HERBALLY YOURS

Enjoy these books!

May your next 40

be healthy!

Toi

1st Printing December 1976
10th Printing January 1979 (Revised)
16th Printing July 1982 (Completely Updated)
20th Printing January 1985
30th Printing August 1989
40th Printing July 1993
45th Printing July 1995
46th Printing February 1996

French Edition:
1st Printing 1977
2nd Printing 1979
3rd Printing 1983
4th Printing 1989
5th Printing 1993

Spanish Edition:
1st Printing 1980
2nd Printing 1987
3rd Printing 1991
4th Printing 1993
5th Printing 1994

Published by:
SOUND NUTRITION
P.O. Box 55
Hurricane, Utah 84737

ISBN # 0–9609226–1–X

TABLE OF CONTENTS

PREFACE

HERBALLY YOURS fills a demand for a comprehensive herbal handbook which is simplified enough for the beginning student and complete enough for the more advanced. It has an alphabetical list of Common Herbs, Health Problems, and some of the most popular Herbal Formulas being used today. There is a chapter on Diet and Cleansing, a brief section on Pregnancy, Nursing and Babies; and a list of Poisonous Herbs and Cautions. Also included is a chapter on Herbal Aid for Emergencies, and Directions on how to make and use herbal preparations such as poultices and tinctures. This book should answer most of your questions about natural health care for you and your family.

The author does not directly or indirectly dispense medical advice or prescribe the use of herbs as a form of treatment for sickness without medical approval. Nutritionists and other experts in the field of health and nutrition hold widely varying views. It is not the intent of the author to diagnose or prescribe. The intent is only to offer health information to help you cooperate with your doctor in your mutual problem of building health. In the event you use this information without your doctor's approval, you are prescribing for yourself, which is your constitutional right, but the publisher and author assume no responsibility.

Author
Penny C. Royal

INTRODUCTION

Dear Jan,

It was good to receive your letter, but I'm sorry you have had so many health problems. Your letter sounded so much like mine would have sounded several years ago. Perhaps if I share my story with you, it will give you comfort and encouragement.

Remember how carefree, energetic and full of life I was in college, and how I would eat anything I desired and never gain a pound? You always said, "Everyone has to watch their waistline, why don't you?"

Well, I took that same habit with me into my career. When most of the other employees had their roll and drink, I had to have creme pies and rich pastries. They were all so envious of me. But Jan, not one of them would envy me in the least had they seen me several years ago — it all caught up with me.

After receiving my immunization shots before going to Europe in 1962, I became very sick. I just assumed that everyone had the same reaction. By the time I arrived in France a month later, I was miserable and in so much pain, I literally could not carry my own purse.

After three months trying to ignore and bear the pain, I had to return home, only to find that my body ws full of Rheumatoid Arthritis. This crippling disease is often brought on by stressful situations and settles in the weak areas of the body. In my case, the shots and foreign travel were more stress than my body could handle. It settled in my back, which was weak from a childhood injury. In any case, I was in pretty bad shape. This was the only time in my life I was considered "fat." I had gained 50 pounds and had that puffy, blown-up look.

After I returned home and received treatment from numerous doctors, and received very little encouragement, I decided I would just have to live with the pain. Since I was unable to return and teach school because of the frequent pain, and my inability to grasp a pencil or chalk, I finally got a job as a receptionist. I sat on a "donut pillow" with a heating pad at my back. It wasn't too bad as I fixed a fancy cover for my pillow and made a pocket in the back of my chair for the heating pad. In this manner I endured the situation while always seeking out any new doctor whom I thought might give me some relief.

About a year and a half later, I met my husband and :ve were married. When I started out with my first pregnancy, I had a very difficult time. I got Bell's palsy, then Pneumonia, which lasted about two months. My delivery was very difficult. I didn't realize just how serious things were until I learned that the doctor slept just outside

5

my room that first night. Also, I spent three days in the recovery room. It did seem rather strange that I had so many roommates during that time. Since the doctor wanted me to see my baby before I died, they brought her to me in the recovery room, which I learned later didn't happen too often. I had to have a blood transfusion and later realized this was when I got Hypoglycemia, or low blood sugar. At that time most doctors weren't too familiar with this disease. It wasn't generally known that diet had anything to do with that particular health problem. I continued to eat the sweets my body craved which gave me a temporary pick-up and when my sugar dropped, I'd just take another goodie. Little did I realize the damage I was causing to my adrenal glands and liver.

Some two years later, during my second pregnancy, I again got Pneumonia and it lasted for 5 months. I had three doctors trying to figure out why my body rejected the antibiotics. They put me in and out of the hospital, but to no avail.

It was during this time that I had numerous problems with constipation and frequent pains in the colon area. The doctor diagnosed it as a nervous colon, then colitis, and finally diverticulitis. By this time, I knew things were getting pretty bad, so I made another appointment with a new clinic. At the end of six hours of testing and examinations by very competent internists, I was told that there was nothing very seriously wrong with me. I did have a slightly overactive thyroid, my blood was low, but in the normal range, I had a cyst on my ovary, but the doctor said it should be watched and possibly would go away without surgery. As for the pains in my colon, well, they wanted to do exploratory surgery and see what was going on inside. My strep throat was still a mystery. You can imagine how I felt as I left the clinic that day.

It was that night I walked the floor asking my Heavenly Father for help. I was guided to a lady who believed in herbs and diet and cleansing. I thought she was "something else," but since I had no other way to go, I followed her diet of raw juices. It was hard for me to suddenly give up all meat and animal products, and I didn't think I could ever exist without my sweets and pastries. I could have only fruits, vegetables, seeds and nuts. My body was so emaciated that it was very difficult to change so suddenly. I couldn't even think clearly — you know the feeling — fuzzy in the brain. I cried a lot and prayed more than I ever had. No one seemed to understand. My own family and friends ridiculed and teased me for the drastic change I had made in diet and cleansing. They knew I would be gone in a short time if I didn't get to a "good doctor." Thanks to an understanding husband, I was able to endure and keep trying. This lady gave me steam baths, and salt scrubs to try and open up my pores. She even gave me enemas to try to clean out the toxins from my system. You see, I didn't realize what I was doing to my body all of those years while I was enjoying my "junk food."

6

I finally reached the point, after three months, that I wanted to try things on my own. It was then that I got the flu and it really hit me hard. Now I realize that it could have been a cleanse that my body was experiencing. Somehow, I remembered a friend telling me about a masseur therapist who had helped her by suggesting only one herb. I had disregarded the story until I lay in bed so very ill. My husband called this therapist and after convincing him that I couldn't even make it to his office, he stopped by our home about 10:30 that evening. He put me on a coffee table in my living room and gave a massage that I shall never forget. Later he told me he had never expected me to pull through the night, so he gave me everything he had. I was black and blue for some time after his treatment, but mighty grateful. Later, I learned that he didn't make house calls. I owe so much to this man, as he literally saved my life. He taught me how to use the herbs and how to live my diet.

I am so grateful for the health I now enjoy and the strength I have been blessed with, so I may in return help others. Even though I still experience bad days, the good ones are more numerous, and the bad ones less frequent. I realize that the body has to back track in order to heal, and the more I study, the more of a miracle I feel it is.

I no longer crave sweets, my body seems to crave things that are good and healthy. I even like vegetables that I didn't even know existed. We keep our meals simple and eat half as much and feel twice as good. I'm so grateful that my husband and children have accepted this change. Oh, I still cheat occasionally, but not too often because I end up paying for it.

Jan, I am no doctor and I can't prescribe or diagnose, but when you reach a point that your body rejects antibiotics, you learn other ways. Please accept the things I have learned and I know you too can experience good health once again.

Since I detest the taste of herb tea, I have had the most experience with capsulated herbs. That doesn't necessarily mean that they are the best, but I found that if I drink plenty of water with them, I get fantastic results. I also know that certain combinations of herbs help specific problems. One person may utilize three out of six while another may use three different ones.

Herbs were put here for our use and I would like to share with you several of my favorite scriptures which kept me encouraged in my search for health.

Genesis 1:29-30
"And God said, behold, I have given you every herb bearing seed, which is upon the face of all the earth, and every tree, in the which is the fruit of a tree yielding seed; to you it shall be for meat.

"And to every beast of the earth, and to every fowl of the air, and to everything that creepeth upon the earth, wherein there is life, I have given every green herb for meat: and it was so."

Doctrine & Covenants, Section 89:10-11

"And again, verily I say unto you, all wholesome herbs God hath ordained for the constitution, nature, and use of man—

"Every herb in the season thereof, and every fruit in the season thereof; all these to be used with prudence and thanksgiving."

Doctrine & Covenants Section 42:43

"And whosoever among you are sick, and have not faith to be healed, but believe, shall be nourished with all tenderness, with herbs and mild food, and that not by the hand of an enemy."

Anyone who is sincerely searching can learn just what is best for his body and in what quantity. And now, after changing my way of life, I no longer suffer from Arthritis, Migraine Headaches, or Strep Throat. My Hypoglycemia is under control, only occasionally do I suffer from Hemmorrhoids. I haven't had Pneumonia for several years. It is wonderful to think clearly once again. I enjoy being alive!

Now, Jan, knowing how much it will mean to you, I dedicate this book to you and many others who are sincerely searching for health, vitality, and a new way of life — through proper diet, herbs, rest, exercise, cleansing, good water, and a healthy mental attitude — and to all of those who have devoted their life to helping others.

HERBALLY YOURS

PENNY C. ROYAL

Chapter 1
DEFINITIONS AND DIRECTIONS

DECOCTION:
A tea made of the roots and bark.
Use 1 Tablespoon of the cut herb or 1 teaspoon of the powdered herb. Gently boil in one cup of water for 30 minutes. Let stand 10 minutes.

EXTRACT:
Extracts are liquid solvents into which the principal ingredients of herb powders are soluble.
The herb powder is put through a special cold extraction process, which calls for cold percolation of the herb with suitable solvents for each herb. Alcohol, water, grape brandy, and apple cider vinegar are the solvents used either singly or in combination.
This percolation with the solvents eventually exhausts the herb of its nutrient factors, active organic properties, organic trace minerals, and enzymes.
Extracts are the result of this process.
Because extracts are in a liquid form they are assimilated, or absorbed into the body much faster. Extracts are used for those who have difficulty in swallowing capsules, and also for small children.

FOMENTATION:
A cloth wrung out of hot infusion or decoction and applied to the affected area. This is usually not as effective as a poultice.

INFUSION:
A tea made of the leaves and blossoms.
Use 1 teaspoon of the powdered herb. Bring 1 cup of water to boiling. Remove from heat. Add the herb. Cover and steep for 10 minutes.

OIL OF HERBS:
An extraction of the herb in an oil base.
Place the powdered herb in the top of a double boiler. Cover with olive oil. Cook on low heat for 3 to 3½ hours. Extract the oil from the mixture. Bottle in dark glass bottles.

POULTICE: *A moist, hot herb pack applied locally.*
                   If using the fresh herb, crush and bruise it.
                   The powdered herb may be used also. Mix
                   with mineral water (or other liquid) to form a
                   thick paste. Spread on a clean cloth and cover
                   the affected area. Leave on for several hours.
                   Always use a fresh poultice. Never re-heat to
                   use over.

TINCTURE: *An extraction of herbs in vinegar or alcohol.*
                   Apple Cider Vinegar is all right for most herbal
                   tinctures. If the herb is oily or sticky, Everclear
                   Brand 190 Proof alcohol can be used
                   successfully.

COMMON TINCTURES

ANTISPASMODIC   Place herbs in 1 quart of Brandy.

    1 oz. Lobelia
    1 oz. Skullcap
    1 oz. Skunk Cabbage
    1 oz. Myrrh
    1 oz. Black Cohosh
    ½ oz. Cayenne

B & B   Place herbs in 1 pint 190 proof alcohol.

    1 oz. Black Cohosh
    1 oz. Blue Cohosh
    1 oz. Blue Vervain
    1 oz. Lobelia
    1 oz. Skullcap

Use for earache, epilepsy, hiccoughs, and muscle spasms.

LOBELIA   Place in 1 pint Apple Cider Vinegar.

    4 oz. Lobelia

Add the herbs to the vinegar or alcohol. Let set for 14 days, shaking 2
or 3 times each day. On the 14th day strain and filter it. If left longer it
goes weak. Place in dark glass bottles.

COMMON EXTRACTS

BLACK WALNUT EXTRACT

Apply topically for Ringworm, Poison Ivy, Poison Oak, and other Skin Problems. Taken internally for Parasites — often combined with #7.

CAYENNE EXTRACT

May be used whenever Cayenne is recommended. For Shock and Hemorrhaging, it is more easily assimilated and works faster than powder.

GINSENG EXTRACT

Older people enjoy this extract because it is easier to take and more rapidly assimilated. Especially good for Senility, Longivity, Energy, and Memory.

HAWTHORN EXTRACT

Used for Heart Ailments.

LICORICE EXTRACT

This extract gives a quick pick-up and is used for those with Hypoglycemia.

LOBELIA EXTRACT

Most relaxing herb. Used in water for small children and applied on body to help relax.

COMBINATION "C"

Chickweed, Black Cohosh, Golden Seal, Lobelia Skullcap, Brigham Tea, Licorice.

Helps to fight infection in the body. Used in the ears and taken internally for Sore Throat and other infections in the body.

COMBINATION "V"

Valerian, Anise, Lobelia, Brigham Tea, Black Walnut, Licorice, Ginger.

Often referred to as the Antispasmodic Herb Combination for Nervous Disorders.

COMBINATION "DQ"

Don Quai, Royal Jelly

Don Quai is the "Queen of the Female Herbs" Royal Jelly is taken from the "Queen" Bee. Very beneficial for skin problems related to Hormone Imbalance in females.

COMMON POULTICES

Fresh: Crush the fresh herb and mix with enough water to make a thick paste, apply to affected area. Put cloth over wound. Change as it dries out. (Plastic may be used to hold moisture in.)

Dried: Mix herb with cornmeal, Slippery Elm, or flax-seed to make thick paste. Add enough boiling water to hold together. Spread on cloth and apply to affected area. Cover and use plastic to hold in moisture.

BAYBERRY
Cancerous sores, Ulcerated sores.

COMFREY
Burns, Sprains, Wounds.

LOBELIA and MULLEIN
Lumps, Lymph Congestion, Swellings.
1 part Lobelia to 3 parts Mullein.

LOBELIA and SLIPPERY ELM
Abecesses, Bites, Blood Poisoning, Boils, Rheumatism, Wounds.
1 part Lobelia to 2 parts Slippery Elm.

ONION
Boils, Sores, Tonsillitis, Ears, Infection.
Use the whole onion which has been heated in oven for earache. Place it against ear to help draw infection out. The onion should be chopped and heated for poultice.

Formula #26
Boils, Burns, Cuts, Wounds.
Mix herbs with either vitamin E or mineral water to make paste. Apply vitamin E on wound before applying paste. Change daily.

PLANTAIN
Blood Poisoning, Dog Bites.

POKE ROOT
Caked Breasts.

POTATO
Growths, Infection, Tumors.
Grate a raw red potato and add 1 teaspoon ginger. Can be used for internal cysts also.

SLIPPERY ELM
Sores, Wounds, Pleurisy.
Excellent mixed with other herbs.

WHITE OAK BARK & GOLDEN SEAL
Varicose Veins, Hemorrhoids.
Equal parts of the two herbs.

CONCENTRATED HERBS

Concentrated herbs follow the same process as the Extracts but are taken one step further. The extracts are subjected to careful dehydration to remove the moisture content, thus resulting in a solvent-free product.

Concentrated herbs are from 4 to 6 times more potent than the conventional Herb Powder.

Advantages: It is more convenient and more economical to use concentrated herbs because it takes fewer capsules to get the same benefit. Concentrated herbs are utilized faster in the body with very little waste. This is important for those with poor digestive systems. The herbs are more assimable in a shorter length of time.

PARTS OF PLANT USED

Bark — Tough outer covering of plant stem, usually only the innerbark (cambium) portion is used.

Berries — Soft fruit of plant, usually with seeds surrounded by a fleshy pulp.

Bulb — Globular-shaped, underground fleshy leaf-bud.

Flowers — Blossoms; reproductive part of plant with colorful, fragrant, modified leaves, and includes flowerheads, flower clusters, etc.

Fruit — Seed-bearing part of plant produced by transformation (ripening) of the ovary, often having a sweet pulp.

Gum — Plant exudate that is gelatinous when moist, and hardens upon drying.

Herb — Above-ground parts (or portions) of plant.

Hips — False fruits formed from flower receptacles.

Hulls — Outer covering of plant fruits.

Leaves — Foliage of plant; expansion from plant stem that is connected with photosynthesis and food manufacture.

Plant — Whole plant, both overground and underground parts are used; also entire seaplants.

Root — Underground parts of plant, including roots, rhizomes, or creeping stems.

Rootbark — Tough outer covering of root, sometimes only the innerbark (cambium) portion is used.

Seeds — Grains or ripened ovules of plant which are capable of germination.

Tops — Uppermost parts of plant, including the flowerheads or flower clusters, tender leaves, and a portion of the soft stems.

Chapter 2
COMMON HERBS

The herbs are used in capsules or teas unless otherwise indicated. The words in bold type are the ones with which we have had the most experience.

ALFALFA
(Medicago sativa) (herb & leaves)

Allergies	Digestive Disorders	**Morning Sickness**
Anemia	Endurance	Nausea
Appetite (improve)	Energy	**Pituitary Gland**
Arthritis	Flu	Rheumatism
Bad Breath	Fractures	Senility
Blood Purifier	Gout	Teeth
Bursitis	Hay Fever	Ulcers
Colon	Hypoglycemia	Uterus
Cramps	Kidneys	Vitality
Diabetes	Lactation	

Because ALFALFA is deep-rooted, it picks up the **trace minerals** in the soil. It contains eight essential **digestive enzymes** and eight **essential amino acids** of protein. It is very rich in **vitamins** and **minerals** including Vitamin U for **peptic ulcers.** It is used for a blood thinner, and a kidney cleanser. Athletes use this herb for endurance & energy.

ALOE VERA
(Aloe species) (leaves)

Abrasions	**Constipation**	Mouth Sores
Acne	Digestive Disorders	Poison Ivy—Oak
Appetite (improve)	Ear Infection	Psoriasis
Athlete's Foot	Eczema	Tonsillitis
Burns	Fractures	Uterus
Cankers	Hemorrhoids	Worms
Colon	Liver	**Wounds**

Aloe Vera is good for chronic constipation—especially in older people. Excellent used as a douche for vaginal discharge and irritation. Especially good for acid burns. It contains allantoin which gives it its healing properties.

CAUTION: For burns, make sure the preparation does *not* contain lanolin, as this will intensify the burn. Aloe Vera should not be taken during the first 3 months of pregnancy. Aloe Vera needs to be stabilized in order to retain its active properties.

BARBERRY

(Berberis vulgaris) (Root Bark)

Anemia
Appetite (improve)
Arthritis
Bladder
Blood Pressure (High)
Blood Purifier
Boils
Colon
Constipation
Diarrhea
Digestive Disorders
Douche
Fever
Gall Bladder
Gall Stones
Gas
Gums
Heart
Heartburn
Jaundice
Kidneys
Liver
Mouth Sores
Rheumatism
Skin Problems
Sore Throat
Spleen
Vagina

Barberry improves the appetite by promoting bile secretion. It will help eliminate gas when used with one part Wild Yam. It has also been used for High Blood Pressure as it dilates the blood vessels. The tea is used as a mouth wash. A low dose stimulates the heart muscle.

CAUTION: A high dose slows down the heart muscle and also the respiratory system and could possibly constrict the broncial tubes.

BAYBERRY

(Myrica cerifera) (Root Bark)

Canker
Childhood Diseases
Circulation
Colds
Colon
Cuts
Diarrhea
Digestive Disorders
Eyes
Fever
Gargle
Hay Fever
Hemorrhage
Hoarseness
Leucorrhea
Lumbago
Lungs
Menstruation (dec)
Miscarriage
Mucous Membranes
Sinus Congestion
Sore Throat
Thyroid (low)
Ulcers
Uterus (prolapsed)
Varicose Veins
Wounds

Bayberry is an astringent and tonic. Helps stop bleeding from lungs, uterus, and colon. Can be used as a poultice for external sores, and the powder can be used as a snuff for nasal congestion & sinus problems. The tea is used as a gargle for sore throat. It improves circulation.

CAUTION: Large doses could cause nausea or vomiting.

BEE POLLEN

(Polen grandular) (Pollen)

Allergies
Asthma
Endurance
Energy
Hay Fever
Hypoglycemia
Longevity
Prostate gland
Vitality

Because of its nutritive value, it is a good source of quick energy. For allergies, start with small doses and gradually build up to large doses as the body builds up a resistance to the allergen.

BISTORT
(Polygonum bistorta) (Root)

Acne
Bed Wetting
Bleeding
Diarrhea
Douche

Gums
Hemorrhage
Insect Bites
Menstruation (dec)
Skin problems

Mouth Sores
Ulcers
Vagina
Worms
Wounds

Bistort is an astringent. It has been used for a mouthwash and gargle, for gum sores, inflammation of the mouth, and sore throat. It helps stop bleeding. It expels worms from the body.

BLACK COHOSH
(Cimicifuga racemosa) (Root)

Arthritis
Asthma
Bee Stings
Blood Pressure (high)
Blood Purifier
Bronchitis
Circulation
Convulsions
Cramps
Coughs
Diabetes

Diarrhea
Epilepsy
Headaches
Heart
Hormones (female)
Hot Flashes
Insect Bites
Kidneys
Liver
Lumbago

Lungs
Menopause
Menstruation (inc)
Nervous Disorders
Rheumatism
Skin Problems
Smoking
Snake Bites
Thyroid
Uterus

Black Cohosh is good for almost all female problems. It is a natural supplier of **estrogen.**

CAUTION: If headaches occur while taking this herb, the body probably has sufficient estrogen and the herb should be discontinued. Herbs containing Progesterone such as Sarsaparilla and Ginseng may be used.

BLACK WALNUT
(Julgans nigra) (Hulls, Leaves)

Boils
Cold Sores
Diarrhea
Douche
Eczema
Lactation (bark)

Leucorrhea
Mouth Sores
Parasites
Poison Ivy
Poison Oak
Ringworm

Skin Rashes
Teeth
Vagina
Venereal Disease
Worms

Black Walnut has been used successfully in a tincture or extract for Poison Ivy, Ringworm, and other types of Skin Problems. It may also be used as a poultice or taken internally. The powder may be used for brushing the teeth to help restore the enamel. When this herb is taken with Formula #7, it will kill most parasites in the body.

BLESSED THISTLE
(Cnicus benedictus) (Herb)

Appetite (improve)	Gall Bladder	Leucorrhea
Arthritis	Gas	Liver
Constipation	Headache	Lungs
Digestive Disorders	**Hormones (female)**	**Menstrual Cramps**
Female Problems	Kidneys	Migraine Headaches
Fever	**Lactation**	Urinary Disorders

Blessed Thistle has been used to increase and enrich the milk in nursing mothers. This herb can be used for female problems when Black Cohosh cannot be tolerated. Good for all urinary, pulmonary, and liver disorders. When Blessed Thistle is given to girls before the onset of Puberty, it will help to alleviate future cramping.

BLUE COHOSH
(Caulophyllum thalictroides) (Root)

Bladder Infection	**Cramps**	Leucorrhea
Blood Pressure (high)	Diabetes	**Menstruation (inc)**
Blood Purifier	Douche	Nervous Disorders
Childbirth	Epilepsy	Smoking
Colic	Heart	Vagina
Convulsions	Kidneys	Water Retention

This herb is formerly known as "Lydia Pinkhams." It stimulates the uterine muscle during childbirth. The Pueblo Indians have used it for years to make childbirth easier. If the baby is ready to be born, it will help dilate the cervix.

CAUTION: Large Doses could cause headache, thirst or convulsions. Activated charcoal will help counteract any negative effects.

BRIGHAM TEA
(Ephedra nevadensis) (Herb)

Arthritis	Colds	Menstruation (inc)
Asthma	Fever	Nosebleed
Blood Pressure (low)	Hay Fever	Rheumatism
Blood Purifier	Headache	**Sinus Congestion**
Childhood Diseases	Kidneys	Skin Problems

This herb is an excellent Spring Tonic. It contains ephedrine (adrenalin), which stimulates the Sympathetic Nervous System which may cause nervousness and restlessness in some people.

BUCHU

(Barosma crenata) (Barosma Betulina) (Leaves)

Bed Wetting	Gravel	Rheumatism
Bladder Weakness	Pancreas	Urethral Irritation
Diabetes	Prostate Gland	Venereal Disease

Buchu is excellent for all types of urinary disorders — including infection, irritation, urine retention, and mucous. It is more effective when taken in combination with Uva Ursi.

BUCKTHORN

(Rhamnus frangula) (Bark)

Constipation	Itching	Rheumatism
Gall Stones	Liver	**Skin Problems**
Gout	Parasites	**Warts**
Hemorrhoids	**Perspiration**	**Worms**

Buckthorn is used mainly as a laxative and is not habit forming. If nausea occurs, this indicates the body has had sufficient — discontinue its use.

BURDOCK

(Arctium lappa) (Root)

Acne	Endurance	Nervous Disorders
Allergies	Energy	Obesity
Arthritis	Fatigue	Poison Ivy-Oak
Baldness	Gall Bladder	Psoriasis
Bladder	Gall Stones	**Rheumatism**
Blood Purifier	Gout	**Skin Problems**
Boils	Hay Fever	Sore Throat
Burns	Hemorrhoids	Tonsillitis
Bursitis	Itching	Ulcers
Cankers	Kidneys	Venereal Disease
Childhood Diseases	Liver	Vitality
Cleansing	Lungs	Water Retention
Dandruff	Lymph Glands	Wounds

Burdock is one of the best blood purifiers without causing nausea or irritation. It helps to reduce swelling and deposits in the joints in Arthritis. Used internally and externally for Skin Problems. The burrs are used for Water Retention. The leaves are used externally for Burns, Skin Problems, and Wounds.

The herbs are used in capsules or teas unless otherwise indicated. The words in bold type are the ones with which we have had the most experience.

CAMOMILE

(Matricaria chamomilla)
(Flowers)

Appetite (improve)	Cramps	Insomnia
Asthma	Dandruff	Jaundice
Bladder	Digestive Disorders	Kidneys
Bleeding	Dizziness	Menstruation (inc)
Blood Purifier	Drug Withdrawal	Migraine Headache
Bronchitis	Earache	**Nervous Disorders**
Callouses	Eyes	Pain
Childhood Diseases	Food Poisoning	**Parasites**
Colds	Gas	Spleen
Colic	Headache	Swelling
Colitis	Hemorrhage	Toothache
Colon	Hemorrhoids	**Worms**
Corns	Inflammation	Wounds

Camomile has been used very successfully as a cleanser for those who have used drugs over a long period of time. The tea is good for Digestive Disorders and tones the complete digestive tract. It is used for expelling Worms in children and also as a hair rinse to add lustre to the hair. Large doses act as an emetic without depressing the system. When used externally as a poultice, it has a drawing and cooling effect. It is often used for preventing Migraine Headaches.

CAPSICUM

(See CAYENNE)

CASCARA SAGRADA

(Rhamnus purshiana)
(Bark)

Colon	**Gall Bladder**	**Liver**
Constipation	Gall Stones	Neverous Disorders
Cough	Hemorrhoids	Pancreas
Croup	Jaundice	Spleen
Digestive Disorders	**Laxative**	

Cascara Sagrada is known as "Doans Pills". It is mainly used for Colon related problems. It stimulates secretions of the Liver, Pancreas, and Stomach when taken internally. Use in small but frequent doses. In chronic Constipation, gradually decrease the dose to stimulate the Peristaltic action of the Colon. It should be taken on an empty stomach. As it restores the tone of the bowel it produces a permanent beneficial effect. It is good taken upon retiring as it helps to relax and soothe the system.

CATNIP
(Nepeta cataria) (Herb)

Bronchitis
Childhood Diseases
Colds
Colic
Convulsions
Cramps
Croup
Diarrhea
Dizziness
Fever

Flu
Gas
Headache
Hypoglycemia
Insomnia
Kidney Stones
Menstruation (inc)
Miscarriage
Morning Sickness

Nervous Disorders
Nightmares
Pain
Parasites
Smoking
Stress
Tension
Uterus
Water Retention

Catnip is used to stop Vomiting. The tea is good for Colic in infants. For fever, use the tea as an enema. This enema is soothing and relaxing and helps dislodge congestion in the Colon. Chew the fresh leaves for Toothache. Catnip elevates the mood and gives one a feeling of well-being.

CAYENNE
(Capsicum annuum, Capsicum frutescens) (Fruit)

Acne
Alcoholism
Appetite (improve)
Arteriosclerosis
Arthritis
Asthma
Bleeding
Blood Pressure (reg)
Bronchitis
Childhood Diseases
Circulation
Colds
Colitis
Convulsions
Cough
Cramps
Cuts
Diabetes

Digestive Disorders
Douche
Endurance
Energy
Eyes
Fatigue
Flu
Fractures
Gas
Hay Fever
Heart Stimulant
Hemorrhage
Hemorrhoids
Infection
Jaundice
Kidneys
Lungs
Menstruation (dec)

Migraine Headaches
Miscarriage
Pancreas
Paralysis
Pleurisy
Rheumatism
Sinus Congestion
Shock
Spleen
Sore Throat
Tonsillitis
Ulcers
Vagina
Varicose Veins
Vitality
Wounds
Yeast Infection

Cayenne has been recognized as one of the greatest of all herbs, not only for the entire digestive system, but for the circulatory system as well. It has been known to be an excellent remedy for Hemorrhoids. It helps to regulate the Heart and Blood Pressure. It strengthens the pulse rate while it cleanses the circulatory system. When taken with Ginger, it helps clean out the Bronchial tubes. (Used with garlic it helps lower the Blood Pressure.) When it is used with other herbs, it acts as a catalyst and increases the effectiveness of the other herbs. It is used for those who are in shock. It helps stop internal or external bleeding if taken internally, or if the wound is small, Cayenne may be applied directly to it. Extract of Cayenne is especially good used as a linament for Headaches, Rheumatism, and Muscle Aches. A small amount of powder sprinkled in your shoes in cold weather will keep your feet warm.

CHAPARRAL

(Larrea divaricata, Larrea mexicana) (Herb)

Acne	Cataracts	Obesity
Allergies	Cleansing	Prostate Gland
Arthritis	Cramps	Psoriasis
Asthma	Dandruff	Rheumatism
Baldness	Eyesight	Skin Problems
Blood Purifier	Hay Fever	**Tumors**
Boils	Insomnia	Warts
Bursitis	Kidneys	Wounds
Cancer		

Chaparral is an astringent and is used externally for sores and wounds. When combined with Red Clover it is used to rid the body of Growths and Tumors by Purifying the Blood.

CHICKWEED

(Stellaria media) (Herb)

Acne	Colon	**Obesity**
Allergies	Constipation	Pleurisy
Appetite (decrease)	Diabetes	Psoriasis
Asthma	Frigidity	Rheumatism
Blood Poisoning	Hay Fever	**Skin Problems**
Boils	Hemorrhoids	Sore Throat
Bronchitis	Hoarseness	Sterility
Burns	**Impotence**	Swelling
Cancer	Inflammation	Tumors
Canker	Itching	Ulcers
Circulation	Mouth Sores	Wounds
Cleansing		

Good to stop bleeding and inflammation from Lungs, Bowels, and Stomach. Used as a poultice for Rashes and Sores. High in Vitamin C. Helps liquify and remove mucous from Respiratory Tract. Helps dissolve fat in the body. May be used as an external scrub for Acne.

CHLOROPHYLL

Acne	Diabetes	Lactation
Anemia	Digestive Disorders	**Liver**
Asthma	**Energy**	Menstrual Cramps
Bad Breath	Foot Odor	Mouth Sores
Blood Purifier	Fractures	Sore Throat
Body Odor	Heart	Thyroid Gland
Cleansing	**Hemorrhage**	Tonsillitis
Colon	Hemorrhoids	Ulcers
Deodorizer	Hypoglycemia	

Chlorophyll may be taken internally or in an enema to remove body odors. It is used as a gargle for Sore Throat and Bad Breath. Very high in trace minerals. It has a high Calcium and Iron content. Iron is necessary for glands to receive sufficient oxygen. It helps to replace Calcium lost during Menstruation. It is an excellent Blood Purifier. Produces more milk in Nursing Mothers. It is good for Hemorrhages because it is high in vitamin K which helps coagulate the blood. Liquid Chlorophyll aids the flow of Bile, which in turn acts as an irritant to encourage the Bowel to function properly.

COMFREY   (Symphytum officinale) (Root)

Allergies	Diabetes	Laxative
Anemia	Diarrhea	Leucorrhea
Arthritis	**Digestive Disorders**	Lumbago
Asthma	Eczema	**Lungs**
Bladder	Fatigue	Menstruation (dec)
Bleeding	**Fractures**	**Mucous Membranes**
Blood Purifier	Gall Bladder	Pneumonia
Boils	Gout	Psoriasis
Bronchitis	Gums	Rheumatism
Bruises	Hay Fever	Sinus Congestion
Burns	Headache	Sore Throat
Bursitis	Hemorrhage	Sprains
Colds	Hoarseness	Swelling
Colitis	Infection	Tonsillitis
Colon	Inflammation	Ulcers
Cough	Insect Bites	**Wounds**
Cramps	Kidneys	

Comfrey helps to eliminate bloody Urine. It is high in Potassium, Vitamin A, and Calcium. The allantoin in Comfrey is the same ingredient that is contained in Aloe Vera. It is soothing to the gastrointestinal tract. It acts as a mild laxative. Poultices of comfrey are very beneficial for Wounds, Sprains, Sores, and Inflammations. Helps to heal broken or fractured bones and is often referred to as the "bone-knitter".

CORN SILK   (Zea mays) (Silk)

Bed Wetting	Gout	Urinary Disorders
Bladder	Kidneys	**Uterine Problems**
Bleeding	Pain	Water Retention
Childbirth	Prostate Gland	

Corn Silk helps rid the body of the ammonia odor in the Urine. It is good for chronic Urinary Disorders, and will alleviate painful urination due to Prostate Gland Problems. It reduces Uric Acid build-up. Helps Uterine Contractions in Childbirth. It also slows down bleeding after the baby is born. It will bring the contractions back during Childbirth if the labor stops.

COUCH GRASS   (Agropyron repens) (Herb)

Bladder	**Kidneys**	Jaundice
Blood Purifier	Gout	Liver
Bronchitis	Gall Stones	Parasites
Constipation	Gravel (bladder)	**Water Retention**

Promotes Urination. Especially effective when taken in combination with other herbs.

CRAMP BARK   (viburnum opulus, v. americanum) (Bark)

Cramps	**Menstruation (inc)**	Nervous Disorders
Kidneys	Miscarriage	Urinary Disorders

Helps to prevent Miscarriage. It relaxes the Ovaries & Uterus. Helps alleviate Cramps in limbs during Pregnancy. Will stimulate the Kidneys. It acts as an antispasmodic to the body. Best when used with Wild Yam, Blue Cohosh, Squaw Vine, or Skullcap.

DAMIANA   (Turnera aphrodisiaca) (Leaves)

Female Problems	**Hot Flashes**	Prostate Gland
Frigidity	Longevity	Senility
Hormones (female)	**Menopause**	**Sex Stimulant**

Damiana is recognized as being good for Females generally, and helps to balance Female Hormones. it also helps to stimulate the Pelvic Organs. Increases the Sex Desire.

DANDELION
(Taraxacum officinale) (Root)

Acne
Age Spots
Anemia
Appetite (improve)
Bladder
Blood Pressure (low)
Blood Purifier
Boils
Bronchitis
Cancer
Cleansing
Constipation
Cramps
Diabetes
Digestive Disorders
Eczema
Endurance
Energy
Fatigue
Fever
Flu
Fractures
Gall Bladder
Gall Stones
Gout
Heartburn
Hemorrhage
Hypoglycemia
Insomnia
Jaundice
Kidneys
Liver
Pancreas
Psoriasis
Senility
Skin Problems
Spleen
Tonsillitis
Vitality
Water Retention
Wounds

Dandelion acts as a tonic to the system. It destroys acids in the blood. As it contains organic Sodium, it is very good for Anemia caused by a deficiency of Nutritive Salts, and is recognized as a great Blood Builder and Purifier. It is also effective as a Liver Cleanser. It is very high in Calcium and other Nutrients. It is a gentle laxative and can therefore be used in a tea for babies and children.

DON QUAI
(Angelica sinensis) (Root)

Anemia
Blood Clots
Blood Pressure (high)
Blood Purifier
Bruises
Cleansing
Convulsions
Cramps
Endurance
Energy
Fatique
Female Problems
Hormones (female)
Hot Flashes
Hypoglycemia
Insomnia
Laxative (mild)
Longevity
Lumbago
Menstrual Cramps
Menopause
Nervous Disorders
Skin Problems
Vitality

This herb is used for almost every female problem. Helps backache caused by menstruation. Acts as a mild laxative as it lubricates the intestines. Has been helpful in eliminating dry skin problems by moistening and softening the skin. Helps to dissolve blood clots. Gives nourishment to the brain cells. High in Vitamin E, B[12]

CAUTION: Not recommended during pregnancy. Could cause enlargement of the breasts.

ECHINACEA

(Echinacea angustifolia)
(Brauneria angustifolia) (Root)

Acne	Carbuncles	Mucous
Bad Breath	**Fever**	Prostate Gland
Bee Stings	Gums	Smoking
Bladder Infection	Hemorrhage	Snake Bites
Blood Poisoning	**Infection**	Tonsillitis
Blood Purifier	Insect Bites	Venereal Disease
Boils	**Lymph Glands**	Wounds

Echinacea is one of the best cleansers for the Lymphatic System. Often used with Myrrh.

EUCALYPTUS

(Eucalyptus globulus) (Oil)

Appetite (improve)	Fever	Nervous Disorders
Bronchitis	Insect Repellant	Paralysis
Cancer	**Lungs**	Sinus Congestion
Colon	Migraine Headache	Sore Throat
Cough	Mucous	Ulcers
Croup	Nausea	Uterus

Only administer in small doses. Helps to dilate capillaries for better cirulation making it a good herb for Migraine Headaches. A small amount on the tongue will help to stop Nausea. It is an antiseptic which makes it good for wounds. Mix with olive oil or vitamin E and apply. Often used in combination with other herbs — Essential Oils. One teaspoon of the oil in 1 cup of warm water, rubbed into the skin is a powerful insect repellant. For coughs, it is as effective as Robitussin, one of the best for expelling mucous.

EYEBRIGHT

(Euphrasia officinalis) (Herb)

Allergies	Digestive Disorders	Hay Fever
Cataracts	**Eye Ailments**	Vision
Diabetes	Glaucoma	

Eyebright has been used for all kinds of Eye Ailments and has been known to strengthen the eyes and improve the eyesight. The tea may be used as an eye wash or the herb may be taken internally.

FALSE UNICORN

(Chamaelirium luteum, Helonias dioica) (Root)

Diabetes	Liver	Senility
Digestive Disorders	Longevity	Sterility
Female Problems	Menstruation (inc)	**Uterus (prolapsed)**
Hemorrhage	**Miscarriage**	Vagina

False Unicorn helps tone the Reproductive Organs by strengthening the muscles of the Uterus and has been used for all types of complications of Pregnancy. Reduces pain in Menstrual Cramps.

FENNEL

(Foeniculum vulgare) (Seeds)

Appetite (normalizes)	Eye Wash	Migraine Headaches
Bed Wetting	Fatigue	**Morning Sickness**
Bronchitis	Gall Bladder	Mucous
Colic	**Gas**	Nausea
Convulsions	Gout	Nervous Disorders
Cough	Hoarseness	Obesity
Cramps	Insect Bites	Rheumatism
D.gestive Disorders	Jaundice	Sinus Congestion
Emphysema	Lactation	Vitality
Endurance	Liver	Water Retention
Energy	Menstruation (inc)	

Fennel was used in the olden times to improve eyesight. It is used in a tea for Colic in babies. It normalizes the Appetite . . . increases or decreases as needed. Fennel helps to increase milk for nursing mothers.

FENUGREEK

(Trigonella foenum graecum) (Seeds)

Allergies	Douche	Lungs
Anemia	Emphysema	**Migraine Headaches**
Bronchitis	Eyes	**Mucous Membranes**
Bruises	Fever	Pneumonia
Colds	Flu	Sinus Congestion
Colitis	Frigidity	Sore Throat
Colon	Hay Fever	Ulcers
Cough	**Headache**	Vagina
Diabetes	Heartburn	Water Retention
Digestive Disorders	Hoarseness	

Fenugreek is an Intestinal Lubricant and is healing for sores and ulcers in the Stomach and Intestines. Used as a Poultice for Wounds and Inflammations. Helps expel Mucous from the Sinuses and prevents Migraine Headaches.

GARLIC (Allium sativum) (Bulb)

Appetite (improve)	Croup	Migraine Headaches
Arteriosclerosis	Diaper Rash	Nasal Passages
Bee Stings	Diarrhea	**Parasites**
Blood Pressure (high)	Digestive Disorders	Prostate Gland
Bronchitis	Douche	Rheumatism
Cancer	Emphysema	Ringworm
Childhood Disease	**Fever**	Sinus Congestion
Circulation	**Gas**	Sore Throat
Colds	**Heart**	Ulcers
Colitis	**Infection**	Vagina
Cough	Insect Bites	Warts
Cramps	Liver	**Yeast Infection**

The antibiotic action of Garlic is very similiar to penicillin and just as effective if taken in large enough doses, but only the harmful bacteria are destroyed. Garlic cleanses Cholesterol from the blood stream. It stimulates the Digestive Tract. Used to kill various kinds of Worms and Parasites when taken as an enema or internally. For chronic Bronchitis, use either Garlic or Onion Poultices on the chest. For Yeast Infection blend 1 clove of Garlic in 1 pint of water, strain, add one or more pints of water and use as a douche. Capsuled Garlic can be used (2 capsules to 1 pint water). Garlic is especially good when used with Hawthorn and Cayenne. In combination with Cayenne it lowers the Blood Pressure.

GINGER (Zingiber officinale) (Root)

Bronchitis	Endurance	Nervous disorders
Childhood Diseases	Energy	Paralysis
Colds	Fatigue	Perspiration (produce)
Colitis	**Flu**	Pneumonia
Colon Spasms	**Gas**	Shock
Cough	Headache	Sinus Congestion
Cramps	Hemorrhage	Stomach Spasms
Croup	Lungs	Toothache
Diarrhea	Menstruation (inc)	Vagina
Digestive Disorders	**Morning Sickness**	Vitality
Douche	Nausea	Vomiting (prevents)

Ginger is used as an antacid because it blocks the breakdown of Pepsinogen to Pepsin—pepsin irritates the tissues and causes Peptic Ulcers. Add 3 or 4 tablespoons to bath water and it will help rid the body of waste and toxins by opening the pores. Ginger is especially good for Colon Gas when taken before each meal. It acts as a catalyst to the Pelvic area.

GINSENG

(Panax quinquefolium) (Root)

Acne	Drug Withdrawl	Inflammation
Age Spots	**Endurance**	**Longevity**
Appetite (improve)	Energy	Lungs
Asthma	Fatigue	Menstruation (inc)
Blood Pressure (reg)	Fever	Pituitary Gland
Cancer	Frigidity	Prostate Gland
Colds	Gas	Senility
Constipation	**Hormones (balance)**	**Sex Stimulant**
Convulsions	Hemorrhage	**Vitality**
Cough	Impotence	Whooping cough
Digestive Disorders		

Ginseng strengthens the Endrocrine Glands which include the metabolism of Vitamins and Minerals. It builds vitality and resistance. It contains Steroids similiar to Estrogen. Ginseng helps to regulate the Male Hormones when used with Sarsaparilla. According to studies done in Russia, the high level of Physical, Spiritual, Emotional, and Mental Endurance has been attributed to the widespread use of Ginseng.

GOLDEN SEAL

(Hydrastis canadensis) (Root)

Allergies	Hay Fever	Obesity
Appetite (improve)	**Hemorrhage**	**Pancreas**
Asthma	Hemorrhoids	Prostate Gland
Bad Breath	Hoarseness	Psoriasis
Bladder	**Infection**	Ringworm
Bronchitis	Inflammation	**Sinus Congestion**
Burns	Itching	Skin Problems
Cancer	Kidneys	**Sore Throat**
Cankers	Leucorrhea	Spleen
Childhood Diseases	Liver	Thyroid (low)
Circulation	Lymph Glands	Tonsillitis
Colds	Menstruation (dec)	Ulcers
Colitis	Morning Sickness	Uterine Problems
Diabetes	Mouth Sores	Uterus
Digestive Disorders	Mucous Membranes	Vagina
Douche	Nasal Passages	Venereal Disease
Eye Wash	Nausea	Water Retention
Flu	Nervous Disorders	Wounds
Gall Bladder	**Nosebleed**	

Its antibiotic action is similiar to Tetracycline and Streptomycin. Contains Hydrastine which is the same ingredient contained in Visine. If a person has Hypoglycemia, it is advisable to take Licorice Root when taking Golden Seal. Myrrh may be used in place of Golden Seal.

GOTU KOLA   (Hydrocotyle asiatica) (Herb)

Aging	Fatigue	Pituitary Gland
Blood Pressure (high)	Longevity	Senility
Brain Food	**Memory**	Skin Problems
Endurance	Menopause	**Vitality**
Energy	Mental Fatigue	Water Retention

Gotu Kola is known as the "Brain Food" as it improves the memory and retards the aging process. It is especially good when taken with Ginseng.

HAWTHORN   (Crataegus oxyacanthus) (Berries)

Adrenal Glands	Endurance	Menopause
Angina	**Energy**	Miscarriage
Arteriosclerosis	Fatigue	Nervous Disorders
Arthritis	**Heart**	Poultice
Blood Pressure	**Hypoglycemia**	Rheumatism
Circulation	Insomnia	Vitality
Emotional Stress	Kidneys	Water Retention

Hawthorn regulates both high and low Blood Pressure. It strengthens the muscle and nerve to the Heart. Helps prevent Miscarriage. The fruit has good drawing properties as a Poultice. Hawthorn may cause dizziness if taken in large doses.

HOPS   (Humulus lupulus) (Flower)

Anemia	Hoarseness	Nightsweats
Appetite (improve)	**Insomnia**	Obesity
Bed Wetting	Jaundice	Parasites
Cough	Liver	Rheumatism
Digestive Disorders	Menstrual Cramps	**Sex Depressant**
Earache	Morning Sickness	Toothache
Fever	**Nervous Disorders**	Ulcers
Headache	Nightmares	Water Retention

Hops is a tonic and has a calming effect on the Heart and Nervous System. Slows down the Sex Desire. Contains Lupulin which is a sedative and hypnotic drug. Use externally for Rheumatism, Bruises, Colic, and Skin Rashes.

The words in bold throughout the book are the ones with which we have had the most success.

HORSERADISH   (Cochlearea armoracia) (Root)

Appetite (improve)	Gas	Parasites
Arthritis	Gout	Rheumatism
Asthma	Hoarseness	**Sinus Congestion**
Bladder	**Hypoglycemia**	Skin Problems
Circulation	Inflammation	Spleen
Cough	Liver	Tumors
Diabetes	Lungs	Water Retention
Digestive Disorders	Mucous	Wounds

Horseradish promotes Digestion. Externally it can be applied to Wounds, Old Sores, Swelling, & Tumors as a Poultice. High Vitamin content. Helps reduce Hoarseness in the Larynx. When mixed with Vinegar, it can be applied to the skin to remove freckles. Good for swollen Liver & Spleen. To clear Nasal Passages in Nursing Babies, the fresh herb may be held close to the nose.

HORSETAIL   (Equsetum arvense) (Herb)

Baldness	Fractures	Nosebleed
Bed Wetting	**Hair**	Obesity
Bladder	Heart	Perspiration Odor
Bleeding	Hemorhage	Toothache
Convulsions	Jaundice	Ulcers
Diabetes	Liver	Urinary Disorders
Earache	Lungs	Uterus
Eyes	Menstruation (inc)	Vagina
Feet	Mucous	Water Retention
Fingernails	**Nervous Disorders**	Wounds

Very healing to the Stomach and Intestinal Ulcers because of its astringent action. Tea is used as a Douche. Strengthens the Hair, Fingernails, and Teeth Enamel. It has a high Silica content which helps the body to assimilate Calcium.

HYSSOP
(Hyssopus officinale) (Herb)

Asthma	Diarrhea	Liver
Bee Stings	Digestive Disorders	Lungs
Bladder	Ears	Mucous
Blood Pressure (reg)	Eyes	Nervous Disorders
Blood Purifier	Gall Bladder	Night Sweats
Bruises	Gall Stones	Parasites
Burns	Gas	Perspiration
Childhood Diseases	Hoarseness	Sinus Congestion
Circulation	Inflammation	Skin Problems
Colon	Insect Bites	Sore Throat
Convulsions	Kidneys	Toothache
Cough	Lice	Ulcers

The Bible tells us "Purge me with Hyssop and I shall be clean." It expels Mucous from all parts of the body. Use the tea as a gargle for Sore Throat. Regulates both high and low Blood Pressure. Can be used as a Poultice on Bruises. For Toothache, boil the herb in vinegar and rinse the Mouth. The mold that produces Penicillin grows on Hyssop Leaves.

IRISH MOSS
(Chondrus crispus) (Plant)

Bad Breath	Fractures	**Obesity**
Cancer	**Goiter**	Pneumonia
Cough	Jaundice	**Thyroid**

Because of the high Iodine content, it is especially good for the Thyroid. Good for Respiratory Tract.

JUNIPER
(Juniperus communis) (Berries)

Adrenal Glands	Blood	Insect Bites
Allergies	Boils	Kidneys
Appetite (improve)	Bronchitis	Lumbago
Arteriosclerosis	Cough	Mucous
Arthritis	**Diabetes**	Pancreas
Baldness	Diuretic	Prostate Gland
Bed Wetting	Gas	Sore Throat
Bee Stings	Hay Fever	Urinary Disorders
Bladder	**Hypoglycemia**	Water Retention

Juniper helps dilate the Bronchial Tubes — it is an antiseptic. Juniper Berries are especially helpful in all Urinary Problems One of the best Diuretics known. Can be used as a disinfectant. Excellent for prevention of Disease. Tea of the berries can be used on Insect Bites & Bee Stings.

31

KELP

(Macrosytic pyrifere) (Plant)

Adrenal Glands	Fractures	**Obesity**
Anemia	**Goiter**	**Pituitary Gland**
Arteriosclerosis	Hot Flashes	Pregnancy
Bursitis	Hypoglycemia	Prostate Gland
Childbirth	Kidneys	Psoriasis
Colitis	Menopause	Skin Problems
Cramps (leg)	Morning Sickness	**Thyroid**
Diabetes	Nausea	Weight Distribution
Eczema		

Especially good for the Adrenal and Pituitary Glands. As it is a natural Iodine, it helps to take weight off the hip area. Repeated small doses will decrease breast milk in Nursing Mothers.

CAUTION: If kelp is not needed, headaches could occur. Often it can be tolerated when taken in combination with other herbs.

LICORICE

(Glycyrrhiza glabra) (Root)

Addison's Disease	**Drug Withdrawal**	Menopause
Adrenal Glands	Emphysema	Mucous Membranes
Age Spots	**Endurance**	Pancreas
Arthritis	Energy	Pneumonia
Asthma	Female Problems	Senility
Blood Purifier	**Hoarseness**	Sex Stimulant
Bronchitis	**Hypoglycemia**	**Sore Throat**
Colds	Laryngitis	Tonic
Constipation	Longevity	Ulcers
Cough	Lungs	**Vitality**

The tea is used for Laryngitis and will restore the Voice. It is also good for a mild laxative for babies. Licorice helps expel Mucous from Respiratory Tract. It contains Estroil, an Estrogen. It contains Nutritive and Laxative Properties. Licorice depresses the Pituitary. It is 50 times sweeter than sucrose and can be used to disguise the taste of bitter herbs. It is one of the most active herbs.

CAUTION: Taken over a long period of time, or in large doses, it can cause sodium and water retention which elevates the blood pressure and may cause pains in the Heart. Listen to your body.

LOBELIA

(Lobelia inflata) (Herb)

Allergies	Fever	Mucous membranes
Arthritis	Food Poisoning	**Nervous Disorders**
Asthma	Hay Fever	**Pain**
Boils	Headache	Pleurisy
Bronchitis	Heart Palpitations	Pneumonia
Bruises	Hoarseness	Poison Ivy—Oak
Bursitis	Hyperactivity	Poultice
Childhood Diseases	Hypoglycemia	**Relaxant**
Cleansing	Insect Bites	Rheumatism
Congestion	Insomnia	Ringworm
Convulsions	Jaundice	Shock
Cough	Liver	Teething
Croup	Lungs	Toothache
Digestive Disorders	Migraine Headaches	Wounds
Ear Infection	Miscarriage	

Lobelia is the most powerful relaxant of all herbs. It should be taken with a stimulant herb such as Cayenne or Peppermint. Lobeline is an alkaloid and is the only active ingredient in Lobelia. Because of the Lobeline's cross tolerance to nicotine, smokers may require more Lobelia. It increases the heart rate, Pituitary function, the Respirations and Peristaltic Movement.

Small doses act as a stimulant. Large doses act as a relaxant. Too much of this herb will cause vomiting.

Use the extract as a rub for relaxing a fretful baby . . . apply on spine. Tincture or extract of Lobelia is used for Croup, Asthma, Earache, Lock Jaw, and Ringworm.

CAUTION: Sometimes it will slow down the body functions. Should not be used by those prone to Diabetes.

MANDRAKE

(Podophyllum peltatum) (Root)

Colitis	**Gall Bladder**	**Laxative**
Constipation	Gall Stones	Liver
Fever	Jaundice	Warts

This herb is very strong and is best used with other herbs in combination.

CAUTION: Use in small amounts.

MARSHMALLOW (Althea officinalis) (Root)

Allergies	Emphysema	Laryngitis
Asthma	Eye Wash	**Lungs**
Bed Wetting	Flu	Menstruation (dec)
Bladder	Hay Fever	Mucous Membranes
Bleeding (Urinary)	Hemorrhage	Nervous Disorders
Burns	Hoarseness	Pain
Cough	Hypoglycemia	Pneumonia
Diabetes	Inflammation	Sore Throat
Diarrhea	**Kidneys**	**Urinary Disorders**
Douche	**Lactation**	Vagina

Because of its mucilaginous properties, it is very soothing and healing. Beneficial in removing stones and gravel from the Urinary Tract and also Hemorrhage from the Urinary Organs. Used as a poultice for Sprains. To increase the flow of milk and make it richer, take as a warm tea.

MISTLETOE (Viscum album) (Herb)

Asthma	Gall Bladder	Hypoglycemia
Blood Pressure (high)	Heart	**Menstruation (dec)**
Convulsions	**Hemorrhage**	Nervous Disorders

Mistletoe is used as a nervine and anti-spasmodic. It will stop Hemorrhage from the Uterus after Childbirth or Miscarriage. It increases the Uterine contractions. It will help expel retained Placenta in childbirth.

CAUTION: This herb should be used with caution as it may cause abortion if taken in large doses. It is used when other herbs fail to stop hemorrhage in Childbirth.

MULLEIN (Verbascum thapsus) (Leaves)

Asthma	**Diarrhea**	Mucous Membranes
Boils	Earache	Nosebleed
Bronchitis	Eyes	Pleurisy
Bruises	Fever	Pneumonia
Bursitis	Glands (swollen)	Poison Ivy —Oak
Childhood Diseases	Hay Fever	**Sinus Congestion**
Colon	**Hemorrhage****	Skin Problems
Constipation	Hemorrhoids	Sore Throat
Cough	Hoarseness	Toothache
Croup	Insomnia	Tumors
Diaper Rash	**Lungs**	Warts

**Will stop Hemorrhage from Bowel and Lungs when taken internally. Use as a tea for Asthma, Diarrhea (enema), and Bleeding from

Bowels. Boil in milk for Cough and Diarrhea. Take in Extract or Tea for Bronchial Problems. Apply as a poultice for Swollen Glands, Stiff Neck, and Mumps. Flowers steeped in oil is a good ointment for Bruises and Frostbite. Apply bruised leaves for Diaper Rash.

MYRRH
(Commiphora Myrrha) (Gum)

Asthma	Digestive Disorders	Nervous Disorders
Bad Breath	Douche	Shock
Blood Purifier	Gums	Sore Throat
Boils	Hypoglycemia	Teeth (stained)
Cankers	Infection	Thrush
Childbirth	Leucorrhea	Thyroid (low)
Colitis	Lungs	Toothache
Colon	Menstrual Cramps	**Ulcers**
Cough	**Mouth Sores**	Vagina
Cuts	Mucous	Wounds

It is an antiseptic which makes it good for Sores and Wounds. For Throat and Mouth Sores, use as a Gargle and Mouthwash. Extract is used for inflammed Gums, Canker, and Thrush. Taken interally helps Bad Breath. Helps to prevent or clear up Infection. In Emergency Childbirth, it can be applied to the navel after the cord is removed. It is used in place of Golden Seal for those with Hypoglycemia.

NETTLE
(Urtica dioica) (Leaves)

Asthma	Diarrhea	Leucorrhea
Baldness	Hemorrhage	Lymph Glands
Bleeding	Insect Bites	Night Sweats
Dandruff	Kidneys	Urinary Problems

Nettle helps expel gravel and stones from any organ where formed—especially the Kidneys.

OAT STRAW
(Avena Sativa) (Stems)

Appetite (improve)	**Fingernails**	Liver
Arthritis	Gall Bladder	Lumbago
Bed Wetting	Gout	Lungs
Bladder	**Hair**	Nervous Disorders
Boils	Heart	Pancreas
Bursitis	Jaundice	Paralysis
Eyes	Kidneys	**Rheumatism**

Oat Straw is very high in Silica and helps the body assimilate Calcium. It is especially good when used with other herbs. It helps to build strong Fingernails, and eliminates split ends of the Hair.

PAPAYA
(Carica papaya) (Fruit)

Allergies	Gas	Parasites
Colitis	Liver	Worms
Digestive Disorders	Mucous Membranes	Wounds

Papaya contains Papain which is an enzyme similar to Pepsin—one produced by the Stomach. Papaya can be mixed with cows milk to resemble breast milk. It has one of the highest enzyme contents of any herb.

PARSLEY
(Petroselinum sativum) (Leaves)

Allergies	Digestive Disorders	Lactation
Appetite (improve)	Eyes	Liver
Arthritis	Fever	Lumbago
Asthma	Fractures	Menstrual Cramps
Bad Breath	Gall Bladder	Menstruation (inc)
Bed Wetting	Gall Stones	Pituitary Gland
Bee Stings	Gout	Prostate Gland
Blood Pressure (low)	Hay Fever	Spleen
Bruises	Insect Bites	Thyroid
Cancer	Kidneys	**Water Retention**
Cough		

Helps Arthritic Pain because of the High Nutritive value. Will bring down a Fever. Parsley will dry up Mother's Milk after Childbirth. Bruised leaves steeped in vinegar and worn next to the breasts will relieve swollen breasts. Parsley helps take away odors on breath from Garlic or other strong herbs. One of the best Diuretics.

PASSION FLOWER
(Passiflora incarnata) (Herb)

Alcoholism	Fever	Insomnia
Blood Pressure (high)	Headache	**Menopause**
Convulsions	**Hot Flashes**	**Nervous Disorders**

When Headaches are caused by Nervous Conditions, this herb will help. In Asthma caused by stress, Passion Flower is very beneficial.

PEACH
(Prunus persica) (Bark)

Bladder	****Morning Sickness**	**Vomiting**
Insomnia	**Nausea	**Water Retention**
Laxative	**Nervous Disorders	Wounds

**For these conditions, the Leaves are used. Peach is best used for a diuretic and a mild laxative.

PENNYROYAL (Hedeoma pulegioides) (Herb)

Burns
Childbirth
Colds
Colic
Convulsions
Cramps

Gout
Headache
Itching
Lungs
Menstruation (inc)
Mucous

Nervous Disorders
Skin Problems
Sore Throat
Toothache
Ulcers
Uterus

Used as a Poultice on Burns. Works on uterine muscle to promote contractions. Contains an oil which relieves headaches if inhaled.

CAUTION: Pennyroyal should not be taken during early Pregnancy as it may cause abortion. At the end of pregnancy, however, it may be used in combination with other herbs to make delivery easier. See Formula #6. It may cause nausea, vomiting, insomnia, disturbed vision if taken in large doses.

PEPPERMINT (Mentha piperita) (Leaves)

Appetite (promotes)
Bronchitis
Childhood Diseases
Colds
Colic
Colitis
Cough
Cramps (stomach)
Diarrhea
Digestive Disorders

Dizzness
Fever
Flu
Gall Baldder
Gas
Headache
Heartburn
Heart Palpatations
Insomnia
Itching

Liver
Menstrual Cramps
Migraine Headaches
Morning Sickness
Muscle Spasms
Nausea
Nervous Disorders
Nightmares
Pain
Smoking

Use in a tea form for all Digestive Disorders. Also, in tea for enemas. Especially good for the Nervous System. Acts as a mild sedative if taken before going to bed. Use in a bath for Itching Skin.

PLANTAIN (Plantago major) (Leaves)

Bee Stings
Bed Wetting
Bladder
Bleeding
Blood Poisoning
Burns
Diarrhea
Douche
Eyes

Fractures
Frigidity
Hemorrhage
Hemorrhoids
Hoarseness
Insect Bites
Itching
Kidneys
Leucorrhea

Lumbago
Lungs
Menstruation (dec)
Poison Ivy-Oak
Thrush
Tumors
Ulcers
Vagina
Wounds

Plantain is used as a poultice on all kinds of Skin Ailments. Rub directly on Rashes caused by Stinging Nettle, Poison Ivy—Oak. Used for Bites, Burns, Rashes, Poisonous Spiders, and Snake Bites.

PLEURISY ROOT

(Asclepias tuberosa) (Root)

Arthritis	Cough	**Pleurisy**
Asthma	Flu	Rheumatism
Bronchitis	**Lungs**	**Pneumonia**
Childhood Diseases	Mucous	Tonsillitis
Circulation	Perspiration (inc)	Water Retention

Pleurisy Root is used to relax the Capillaries. It is used in all Lung-Related Problems

CAUTION: Do not use when skin is cold and pulse is weak.

POKE WEED

(Phytolacca decandra) (Root)

Breasts	**Inflammation**	Rheumatism
Cancer	Laxative	Ringworm
Constipation	Liver	Skin Problems
Goiter	Lumbago	**Thyroid**
Gums	**Lymph Glands**	Tumors
Hemorrhoids	Pain	Ulcers
Infection	Parasites	

For inflammed or swollen Breasts, use internally or as a poultice. Regulates the Thyroid Gland. Should be used in small doses.

CAUTION: May cause Digestive Upset.

PRIMROSE

(Primula vulgaris, P. officinalis) (Seed, Oil)

Arthritis	Gall Stones	Pain
Blood Pressure (high)	Gout	Rheumatism
Bronchitis	Insomnia	Stomach
Convulsions	**Nervous Disorders**	**Toothache**

Primrose acts as a stimulant to the Bronchial Tubes and Stomach. It is an antispasmodic. It neutralizes over-acidity in the body. The root is used to expel worms. Best used in an OIL.

PSYLLIUM

(Plantago psyllium) (Seeds)

Colitis	**Constipation**	Hemorrhoids
Colon	Laxative (mild)	Ulcers

Psyllium helps to lubricate and heal the Intestinal Tract. It also moistens and acts as a bulk agent. It is sold in stores under the name Metamucil.

QUEEN OF THE MEADOW
(Eupatorium purpureum)
(Leaves)

Diabetes	Nervous Disorders	**Urinary Disorders**
Gout	Prostate Gland	Uterus
Kidneys	Rheumatism	Vagina
Lumbago	Stones	**Water Retention**

Used for Bladder & Kidney Problems especially when gravel and stones are present. Used in combination with other herbs.

RED CLOVER
(Trifolium pratense) (Flowers)

Acne	**Cancer**	**Nervous Disorders**
Arthritis	Childhood Diseases	Psoriasis
Blood Purifier	Cleansing	Rheumatism
Boils	Flu	**Skin Problems**
Bronchitis	Insomnia	**Tumors**

This herb has been used to restore fertility. It is a mild Laxative. Especially good to calm the Nerves and cleanse the Blood. It helps to break up Growths and Tumors when used in combination with Chaparral and other herbs.

RED RASPBERRY
(Rubus idaeus) (Leaves)

Afterpain	Eyewash	Mouth Sores
Bronchitis	Female Organs	Mucous Membranes
Canker	**Flu**	Nausea
Childbirth	Fractures	Nervous Disorders
Childhood Diseases	Lactation	Pregnancy
Colds	Leucorrhea	Rheumatism
Constipation	Menstruation (dec)	Sore Throat
Diabetes	Menstrual cramps	Ulcers
Diarrhea	**Morning Sickness**	Uterus
Digestive Disorders		

It strengthens the Uterus and entire Reproductive System therefore, it is good to use during the whole Pregnancy. Coordinates Uterine contractions in Childbirth. It is not a pain-killer — this enables it to cross the Placental Membrane without depressing the Respiratory and Circulatory Centers in the Brain. Decreases chance of Miscarriage for Premature Babies. Helps mother carry baby full term as it decreases contractions in the 2nd Trimester of Pregnancy. For Flu and Diarrhea in Children, take as a tea or use as an enema.

REDMOND CLAY
(Montmorillonite) (Clay)

Acne	**Bee Stings**	**Skin Problems**

Used as a poultice to draw infection from the body. Excellent used in an enema to draw toxins from the Colon. Can be used externally as a poultice for Skin Problems.

ROSE HIPS
(Rosa canina) (Fruit)

Arteriosclerosis	Emphysema	Jaundice
Bee Stings	Fever	Kidneys
Bruises	Flu	Poison Ivy-Oak
Childhood Diseases	Heart	Sinus Congestion
Circulation	**Infection**	Sore Throat
Colds	Insect Bites	Tonsillitis

Excellent source of natural Vitamin C. Used for infection and cleansing toxins from the body.

SAFFLOWER
(Carthamus tinctorius) (Flower)

Appetite (improve)	Gall Bladder	**Liver**
Arthritis	**Gas**	Menstruation (inc)
Bronchitis	**Gout**	Perspiration (inc)
Childhood Diseases	Heart	Psoriasis
Cramps	Heartburn	Sex Stimulant
Digestive Disorders	Hemorrhoids	**Uric Acid**
Fever	Hypoglycemia	**Water Retention**
Frigidity		

Safflower prevents and helps to eliminate the buildup of Uric and Lactic Acid in the body which causes Gout. It alleviates Fatigue and Muscle Cramps after exertion or exercise, especially in those with Hypoglycemia. It is similiar to Camomile in action and uses.

SAGE
(Salvia officinalis) (Leaves)

Baldness	Headache	**Nervous Disorders**
Bleeding	Hoarseness	**Night Sweats**
Bronchitis	Insect Bites	Parasites
Dandruff	**Lactation**	Sex Depressant
Diarrhea	Laryngitis	Skin Problems
Digestive Disorders	Lungs	Sore Throat
Dizziness	Menstruation (inc)	Tonsillitis
Fever	Morning Sickness	Ulcers
Flu	Mouth Sores	**Worms**
Gas	Mucous Membranes	Wounds
Hair	Nausea	

40

Sage contains a volatile oil and is used by dentists to decrease saliva. Tea used as a mouth wash and gargle. Helps to eliminate spasms of the Gastrointestinal Tract. Sage is used to help dry up milk in nursing mothers. Helps rid the body of Worms in children.

SARSAPARILLA
(Smilax officinalis) (Root)

Acne	Frigidity	Mucous
Age Spots	Gout	Psoriasis
Blood Purifier	**Hormones**	Rheumatism
Boils	Heart Burn	Ringworm
Colds	**Hot Flashes**	Senility
Cough	Longevity	Sterility
Eyes	Menopause	Water Retention
Fever		

Sarsaparilla contains Hormones for both male and female. When it is used with Ginseng, it helps to eliminate acne due to hormone imbalance in teenage boys.

SAW PALMETTO
(Serenoa Serrulata) (Fruit)

Alcoholism	Bronchitis	Glands (swollen)
Asthma	Colds	**Hormones**
Bladder	Diabetes	**Obesity**
Breasts	**Frigidity**	Prostate Gland

Saw Palmetto contains the enzyme lipase, which helps break down fat. It helps underweight people to gain weight. It also has been used to help increase the size of small breasts. It acts as a regulator of Weight and also Hormones.

SKULLCAP
(Scutellaria lateriflora) (Herb)

Alcoholism	Digestive Disorders	**Nervous Disorders**
Bed Wetting	Headache	Paralysis
Blood Pressure (high)	Hypoglycemia	Rheumatism
Childhood Diseases	Insect Bites	**Sex Depressant**
Convulsions	**Insomnia**	Smoking

Since Skullcap is an antispasmodic, it is one of the most effective nervous system relaxants. It decreases sex desire.

SPEARMINT
(Mentha viridis) (Leaves)

This herb is used the same as Peppermint but because it is a milder herb, it is often preferred for small children.

SLIPPERY ELM   (Ulmus fulva) (Bark)

Asthma	Douche	Ovaries
Bladder	Eczema	Pleurisy
Boils	Eyes	Sex Stimulant
Bronchitis	Flu	Smoking
Burns	**Fractures**	Sore Throat
Cancer	Hemorrhage	Stomach
Colitis	**Hemorrhoids**	Tapeworms
Colon	Hoarseness	Tonsillitis
Constipation	Inflammation	Ulcers
Cramps	Leucorrhea	Uterus
Cough	Lumbago	Vagina
Diaper Rash	Lungs	Water Rentention
Diarrhea	Mucous Membranes	**Wounds**
Digestive Disorders		

Slippery Elm can be used internally, or externally. Because of its mucilage properties it coats the Digestive Tract and aids in healing inflammation and is very soothing for Ulcers. Blend 1 teaspoon of powder in 1/2 cup water and give orally or in an enema for Diarrhea and Nausea. It can be used as a bolus for Uterine problems. Excellent used as a Poultice and is often mixed with Golden Seal and Comfrey.

SQUAW VINE   (Mitchella repens) (Herb)

Childbirth	Insomnia	Nervous Disorders
Eyewash	**Menstruation (inc)**	

Squaw Vine is an astringent, tonic, and diuretic. It works especially well for Childbirth when combined with Red Raspberry.

ST. JOHNSWORT   (Hypericum perforatum) (Herb)

Afterpain	Gout	Nervous Disorders
Anemia	Heart	Skin Problems
Bed Wetting	Hemorrhage	Ulcers
Bruises	Insect Bites	Urinary Disorders
Burns	Jaundice	Water Retention
Cough	Lungs	Worms
Diarrhea	Menstruation (inc)	Wounds

Used for persistent mucous problems from Lungs, Bowels, and Urinary Tract. Use as poultice for relief of local Pains and Bruises. Helps alleviate afterpain in Childbirth.

STRAWBERRY
(Fragaria vesca) (Leaves)

Anemia	Digestive Disorders	Menstrual Cramps
Appetite (improve)	Fever	Nervous Disorders
Blood Purifier	Gall Bladder	Night Sweats
Bowel Problems	Liver	Vitality

The fruit may be used to cleanse tartar from the teeth and will whiten stained teeth by leaving it on for awhile. The fruit is also good for a facial scrub. The tea of the leaves is used for Eczema, Sore Eyes, and Styes on eyelids. High in minerals.

TAHEEBO
(Tabebuia avellanedae) (inner bark)

Anemia	Hemorrhage	**Rheumatism**
Appetite (improve)	**Herpes Simplex**	Ringworm
Blood Purifier	Insomnia	Skin Problems
Cancer	Kidneys	Ulcers
Cleansing	Leukemia	Varicose Veins
Colon	Nervous Disorders	**Venereal Disease**
Diabetes	**Pain**	Water Retention
Digestive Disorders	Prostate Gland	Wounds
Hemorrhoids		

High in Iron. It is a detoxifier. It puts the body in a defensive state to give it the energy needed to defend itself and to help resist disease. Taheebo is an Indian name for inner bark of Red Lapacho Tree found in the Andes Mountains. It seems to be most effective taken in tea. Especially good for pain connected with Cancer.

THYME
(Thymus vulgaris) (Herb)

Asthma	Eczema	Liver
Bad Breath	Fever	Lungs
Bronchitis	Flu	**Migraine Headache**
Childhood Diseases	Headache	Mucous
Cough	**Heartburn**	Nervous Disorders
Cramps	Hookworms	Nightmares
Diarrhea	Kidney Stones	Parasites
Digestive Disorders	Leucorrhea	Sore Throat

Helps expel Mucous from Digestive, Respiratory and Urinary Tracts. Helps prevent build-up of Kidney Stones. Expels retained Afterbirth. Used with Fenugreek, it prevents Migraine Headaches and clears sinuses.

TURKEY RHUBARB
(Rheum palmatum) (Root)

Anemia	Colon	Hemorrhoids
Appetite (improve)	**Constipation**	Jaundice
Bad Breath	Croup	**Laxative**
Colitis	Headache	Liver

Because it keeps the stool soft, it helps alleviate Hemorrhoids. Acts as a mild Laxative.

UVA URSI
(Arctostaphylos uva ursi) (Leaves)

Appetite (improve)	Hemorrhoids	Pancreas
Bed Wetting	**Kidneys**	Prostate Gland
Bladder	**Kidney Stones**	Spleen
Bronchitis	Leucorrhea	**Urinary Disorders**
Cystitis	Liver	Uterus (prolapsed)
Diabetes	Menstruation (dec)	Vagina
Digestive Disorders	Mucous Membranes	Veneral Disease
Female Problems	Obesity	**Water Retention**

For chronic Urinary Problems, this herb can be safely used on a continuing basis and in high doses.

VALERIAN
(Valeriana officinalis) (Root)

Acne	Epilepsy	Menstruation (inc)
Afterpain	Fever	Migraine Headache
Alcoholism	Gas	**Nervous Disorders**
Blood Pressure (high)	Heart	**Pain**
Childhood Diseases	Heartburn	Paralysis
Colds	Hypoglycemia	Shock
Colic	**Insomnia**	Smoking
Convulsions	Lumbago	Ulcers
Digestive Disorders	Menopause	Wounds

Valerian is very relaxing to the whole system. It will stop headaches due to menopause. Has a tranquilizing effect similar to Valium.

WHITE OAK BARK
(Quercus alba) (Bark)

Acne	Jaundice	**Teeth**
Bladder	Kidneys	**Thrush**
Bruises	**Leucorrhea**	Tonsillitis
Canker	Liver	Toothache
Diarrhea	Menstruation (dec)	**Ulcers**
Douche	**Mouth Sores**	**Urinary Disorders**
Fever	Nose	Uterus (prolapsed)
Gall Bladder	Parasites	Vagina
Goiter	Ringworm	**Varicose Veins**
Hemorrhage	Skin Problems	Wounds
Hemorrhoids	Sore Throat	Yeast Infection

This herb is both an astringent and tonic. Tannic Acid is the active ingredient. White Oak Bark is good to harden the gums prior to the fitting of false teeth. It will set loose teeth and also heal most sores in the mouth. The tea is a good douche for Yeast infection. A cloth wrung out of the tea and applied directly to Varicose Veins helps reduce the size. The herb is used both internally and externally.

WILD YAM
(Dioscorea villosa) (Root)

After Pain	**Morning Sickness**	**Stomach**
Colic	Nausea	Ulcers
Gas	Nervous Disorders	**Uterine Pains**
Menstrual Cramps	Pain	

Wild Yam may be taken during Pregnancy to help eliminate cramps. It relieves gas pains in the Stomach. Relieves Nausea. Prevents Miscarriage. Has been used as a contraceptive. It contains similar properties as the "pill". Contains Steroids.

WILLOW
(Salix) (Bark)

Arthritis	Dandruff	Gums
Baldness	Eyes	**Headache**
Bed Wetting	Fever	Hemorrhage
Burns	Gall Stones	Rheumatism
Bursitis	Gas	Sex Depressant
Convulsions	Gout	Wounds

Contains salicin which is the main ingredient in Aspirin.

The words in bold throughout the book are the ones with which we have had the most success.

WINTERGREEN

(Gaultheria procumbens)
(Leaves-Oil)

Diabetes	Inflammation	Stomach
Digestive Disorders	Leucorrhea	Swelling
Fever	**Pain**	Varicose Veins
Headache	Rheumatism	Venereal Disease
Heart	Skin Problems	Water Retention

Most effective as an oil. Wintergreen contains Salicylic Acid and when combined with Acetic Acid (vinegar) has the same properties as Aspirin . . . making it good for Pain and Headaches. Small doses stimulate the Stomach, Heart, and Respiratory Systems. The tea is used for a gargle for Sore Throat and Mouth and is used in a Douche for Leucorrhea. The oil is used in linaments. Poultices are for Boils, Swellings, and Inflammations. It does not contain any anti-inflammatory properties therefore it is not good for Arthritis and Rheumatism without combining with other herbs. Excellent when used in combination with other "Essential Oils."

WITCH HAZEL

(Hamamelis virginiana) (Bark)

Cuts	**Hemorrhoids**	Sore Throat
Douche	Inflammation	**Varicose Veins**
Eyes	Mucous Membranes	Venereal Disease
Gums	Nosebleed	Wounds
Hemorrhage	Sinus Congestion	

Used as a mouthwash for Bleeding Gums and after tooth extraction. Use the tea or extract as gargle for Sore Throat. Use packs on eyes for bruised or inflamed eyes.

WOOD BETONY

(Betonica officinalis) (Herb)

Asthma	**Headache**	**Nervous Disorders**
Bed Wetting	Heart	**Pain**
Bladder	Heartburn	Parasites
Bronchitis	Inflammation	Perspiration (dec)
Convulsions	Insect Bites	Sprains
Cough	Jaundice	Stomach
Diarrhea	Kidneys	Tonsillitis
Digestive Disorders	Liver	Varicose Veins
Dizziness	**Migraine Headache**	Wounds
Gout	Menstruation (dec)	

Especially good for headaches when taken with Fenugreek and Thyme. It is good to heal old sores. Relaxes the whole system.

YARROW

(Achillea Millefolium) (Flower)

Appetite (improve)	Dandruff	Liver
Arthritis	Diabetes	Lungs
Baldness	Diarrhea	Menstrual Cramps
Bladder	Ear Infection	Mucous Membranes
Bleeding	Female Problems	Nervous Disorders
Blood Purifier	Fever	Night Sweats
Bruises	**Flu**	Perspiration (inc)
Bursitis	Fractures	Pleurisy
Childhood Diseases	Headache	Pneumonia
Colds	**Hemorrhage (lungs)**	**Skin Problems**
Colic	Hemorrhoids	**Sore Throat**
Colon	Insomnia	Spleen
Congestion	Jaundice	Uterus
Cuts	Kidneys	Wounds

Yarrow is good for clearing Mucous discharge from the Bladder. Will produce perspiration by opening the pores. Reduces clotting time so it is good for bleeding if used internally. Contains steroids. Use the tea for a shampoo to help Baldness.

YELLOW DOCK

(Rumex crispus) (Root)

Acne	Ear Infection	Itching
Anemia	**Energy**	**Liver**
Bladder	Eyes	Pancreas
Blood Purifier	Fatigue	Pituitary Gland
Boils	Fever	Poison Ivy-Oak
Cancer	Flu	Psoriasis
Childhood Diseases	Fractures	**Skin Problems**
Cleansing	Gall Bladder	Spleen
Diabetes	Glands (swollen)	Tumors
Digestive Disorders	Gout	Ulcers
Earache	Inflammation	Venereal Disease

Yellow Dock acts as a natural Iron in the system. Especially good as a Blood Purifier and body Cleanser. It is helpful for ulcerated Eyelids. For Itching, use internally or in a bath.

YUCCA

(Yucca baccata) (Root)

Arthritis	Gout	**Rheumatism**
Blood Purifier	Inflammation	Ulcers
Bursitis	Joints	Wounds

The Southwest Indians use it for its Cleansing and Detergent properties. Excellent as a hair shampoo. Yucca contains Steroids therefore it is used to reduce inflammation from the joints.

Chapter 3
HERBAL FORMULAS

For convenience and space, the following Formulas will be referred to throughout the book by the number on the left.

1. ALLERGY, HAY FEVER, & SINUS FORMULAS

_____ A. Black Cohosh, Blessed Thistle, Pleurisy Root, Skullcap.

_____ B. Brigham Tea, Burdock, Cayenne, Chaparral, Golden Seal, Lobelia, Marshmallow, Parsley.

Allergies	Hay Fever	Mucous
Asthma	Insect Bites	Sinus Congestion

2. ARTHRITIS FORMULAS

_____ A. Alfalfa, Black Cohosh, Bromalain, Burdock, Cayenne, Centaury, Chaparral, Comfrey, Lobelia, Yarrow, Yucca.

_____ B. Black Cohosh, Black Walnut, Brigham Tea, Burdock, Cayenne, Chaparral, Hydrangea, Lobelia, Sarsaparilla, Skullcap, Valerian, Wild Lettuce, Wormwood, Yucca.

Arthritis	Gout	Rheumatism
Bursitis	Inflammation	Swelling

3. BLOOD BUILDER FORMULAS

_____ A. Alfalfa, Dandelion, Kelp

_____ B. Burdock, Lobelia, Mullein, Nettle, Red Beet, Strawberry, Yellow Dock.

Anemia	Fatigue	Pregnancy
Blood Builder	Goiter	Senility
Cramps (leg)	Pancreas	Thyroid
Endurance	Pituitary Gland	Water Retention
Energy		

4. BLOOD PURIFIER FORMULAS

_____ A. Barberry, Burdock, Cascara Sagrada, Chaparral, Dandelion, Licorice, Red Clover, Sarsaparilla, Yarrow, Yellow Dock.

_____ B. Buckthorn, Burdock, Cascara Sagrada, Chaparral, Licorice, Oregon Grape, Peach, Prickly Ash, Red Clover, Sarsaparilla, Stillingia.

Acne	Cleansing	Lymph Glands
Age Spots	Colon	Pancreas
Anemia	Constipation	Poison Ivy—Oak
Arthritis	Eczema	Rheumatism
Bad Breath	Fever Blisters	Ringworm
Blood Poisoning	Infection	Skin Problems
Blood Purifier	Inflammation	Spleen
Boils	Insect Bites	Tonsillitis
Cancer	Itching	Tumors
Canker	Jaundice	Veneral Disease
Childhood Diseases	Liver	Wounds

5. CALCIUM FORMULAS

_____ A. Alfalfa, Comfrey, Horsetail, Irish Moss, Lobelia, Oat Straw.

_____ B. Comfrey, Horsetail, Lobelia, Oat Straw.

Afterpain	Fingernails	Nervous Disorders
Allergies	Flu	Nightmares
Arteriosclerosis	Fractures	Obesity
Arthritis	Gout	Pain
Bed Wetting	Hair	Pregnancy
Bursitis	Headaches	Rheumatism
Childbirth	Hypoglycemia	Teeth
Colds	Insomnia	Toothache
Colitis	Joints	Ulcers
Convulsions	Lactation	Varicose Veins
Cramps	Lumbago	Water Retention
Eczema	Migraine Headaches	Wounds

6. CHILDBIRTH FORMULAS

_____ A. Black Cohosh, Lobelia, Pennyroyal, Red Raspberry, Squaw Vine.

_____ B. Hibiscus, Peppermint, Red Raspberry, Rose Hips

Childbirth	Delivery	Hormones (Regulate)

"B" is used during the entire pregnancy in tea form.

7. CLEANSING FORMULAS

_____ A. Barberry, Black Walnut, Catnip, Chickweed, Comfrey, Cyani Flowers, Dandelion, Echinacea, Fenugreek, Gentian, Golden Seal, Irish Moss, Mandrake, Myrrh, Safflower, St. Johnswort, Yellow Dock.

_____ B. Cascara Sagrada, Comfrey, Culver's Root, Mandrake, Mullein, Pumpkin Seeds, Slippery Elm, Violet, Witch Hazel.

Cancer	Constipation	Skin Problems
Cleansing	Parasites	Tumors
Colon	Prostate Gland	Worms

These Formulas work better for Parasites when taken with extra Black Walnut. As these formulas break toxins from the body, it is suggested that enemas be used. (See chapter 8) "B" is specifically used for Parasites and Prostate Gland.

8. COLD FORMULAS

_____ A. Cayenne, Camomile, Golden Seal, Lemon Grass, Myrrh, Peppermint, Rose Hips, Sage, Slippery Elm, Yarrow.

_____ B. Garlic, Parsley, Rosehips, Rosemary, Watercress

Bronchitis	Colds	Flu
Childhood Diseases	Ear Infection	Mucous

9. COLON FORMULAS

_____ A. Barberry, Buckthorn, Cascara Sagrada, Cayenne, Couch Grass, Ginger, Licorice, Lobelia, Red Clover.

_____ B. Barberry, Cascara Sagrada, Cayenne, Fennel, Ginger, Golden Seal, Lobelia, Red Raspberry, Turkey Rhubarb.

_____ C. Comfrey, Pepsin

Acne	Cleansing	Croup
Allergies	Colds	Ear Infection
Asthma	Colitis	Fever
Bad Breath	Colon	Parasites
Bronchitis	Constipation	Sinus Congestion

10. DIABETES & PANCREAS FORMULAS

_____ A. Bistort, Buchu, Cayenne, Comfrey, Dandelion, Garlic, Golden Seal, Huckleberry, Juniper, Licorice, Marshmallow, Mullein, Uva Ursi, Yarrow.

_____ B. Cayenne, Golden Seal, Juniper, Licorice, Mullein, Uva Ursi.

Bladder	Hypoglycemia	Pancreas
Diabetes	Kidneys	Urinary Disorders

11. DIGESTION FORMULAS

_____ A. Alfalfa, Peppermint.

_____ B. Papaya, Peppermint.

_____ C. Catnip, Fennel, Ginger, Lobelia, Papaya, Peppermint, Spearmint, Wild Yam.

Appetite	Cramps (stomach)	Gas
Colic	Digestive Disorders	Heartburn

12. EYE FORMULAS

_____ A. Bayberry, Eyebright, Golden Seal.

_____ B. Bayberry, Cayenne, Eyebright, Golden Seal, Red Raspberry.

Allergies	Eyes	Glaucoma
Cataracts	Diabetes	Hay Fever

13. FEMALE HORMONE FORMULAS

_____ A. Blessed Thistle, Cayenne, Ginger, Golden Seal, Lobelia, Marshmallow, Parsley, Queen of the Meadow, Red Raspberry.

_____ B. Black Cohosh, Blessed Thistle, False Unicorn, Ginseng, Licorice, Sarsaparilla, Squaw Vine.

_____ C. Blessed Thistle, Cayenne, Cramp Bark, False Unicorn, Ginger, Golden Seal, Red Raspberry, Squaw Vine, Uva Ursi.

_____ D. Black Cohosh, Blessed Thistle, Don Quai, Ginger, Licorice, Marshmallow, Queen of the Meadow, Red Raspberry.

Acne	Menopause	Puberty
Female Problems	Menstrual Cramps	Sterility
Frigidity	Obesity	Uterus
Hot Flashes	Pregnancy	Vagina

14. FLU FORMULAS

_____ A. Cayenne, Ginger, Golden Seal, Licorice.

_____ B. Bayberry, Cayenne, Cloves, Ginger, White Pine Bark.

Colds	Flu	Muscle Pains
Cramps (stomach)	Gas	Nausea
Digestive Disorders	Lymph Glands	Sore Throat
Fever	Morning Sickness	Vomiting

15. HEADACHE FORMULAS

_____ A. Fenugreek, Thyme

_____ B. Fenugreek, Passion Flower, Peppermint, Thyme, Wood Betony.

Bronchitis	Fever	Heartburn
Cough	Flu	Migraine Headache
Digestive Disorders	Headache	Sore Throat

16. HEART & BLOOD PRESSURE FORMULAS

_____ A. Cayenne, Garlic, Hawthorn.

_____ B. Cayenne, Garlic.

_____ C. Cayenne, Garlic, Ginger, Ginseng, Golden Seal, Parsley.

Adrenal Glands	Circulation	Heart
Arteriosclerosis	Cholesterol	Shock
Blood Pressure (Reg)	Energy	Varicose Veins

"A" is used to strengthen the Heart, "B" is used for High Blood Pressure, and "C" is used to equalize the Blood Pressure.

17. HYPOGLYCEMIA FORMULAS

_____ A. Dandelion, Horseradish, Licorice, Safflower.

_____ B. Cayenne, Red Clover, Soy Beans.

Adrenal Glands	Energy	Hypoglycemia

18. INFECTION FORMULAS

_____ A. Cayenne, Echinacea, Myrrh, Yarrow.

_____ B. Cayenne, Echinacea, Golden Seal, Yarrow.

_____ C. Black Walnut, Bugleweed, Golden Seal, Lobelia, Marshmallow, Plantain.

_____ D. Chickweed, Black Cohosh, Golden Seal, Lobelia, Skullcap, Brigham Tea, Licorice.

Childhood Diseases	Flu	Pneumonia
Colds	Infection	Sinus Congestion
Ear Infection	Lymph Glands	Sore Throat
Fever	Mucous	Tonsillitis

"D" is best used in an extract, it is for ear infection, sore throat, and other infections in the body.

19. KIDNEY & BLADDER FORMULAS

_____ A. Camomile, Dandelion, Juniper, Parsley, Uva Ursi.

_____ B. Ginger, Golden Seal, Juniper, Lobelia, Marshmallow, Parsley, Uva Ursi.

Bed Wetting	Diuretic	Urinary Disorders
Bladder	Kidneys	Water Retention

20. LIVER & GALL BLADDER FORMULAS

_____ A. Angelica, Birch, Blessed Thistle, Camomile, Dandelion, Gentian, Golden Rod, Horsetail, Liverwort Leaves, Lobelia, Parsley, Red Beet.

_____ B. Barberry, Catnip, Cramp Bark, Fennel, Ginger, Peppermint, Wild Yam.

Age Spots	Gall Bladder	Liver
Cleansing	Gall Stones	Pancreas
Dizziness	Jaundice	Spleen

21. LUNG FORMULAS

_____ A. Comfrey, Lobelia, Marshmallow, Mullein, Slippery Elm.

_____ B. Chickweed, Comfrey, Lobelia, Marshmallow, Mullein.

_____ C. Comfrey, Fenugreek.

Allergies	Emphysema	Mucous
Asthma	Hay Fever	Pleurisy
Bronchitis	Hoarseness	Pneumonia
Cough	Lungs	Sinus Congestion

22. MEMORY FORMULAS

_____ A. Cayenne, Ginseng, Gotu Kola.

_____ B. Bayberry, Bee Pollen, Black Walnut, Cayenne, Comfrey, Eucalyptus, Fennel, Gentian, Ginseng, Ho Shou-Wu, Lemon Grass, Licorice, Myrrh, Peppermint, Safflower.

Drug Withdrawl	Longevity	Senility
Endurance	Memory	Sterility
Energy	Pituitary Gland	Vitality

23. NERVE & SLEEP FORMULAS

_____ A. Black Cohosh, Cayenne, Ginger, Hops, Mistletoe, St. Johnswort, Valerian, Wood Betony.

_____ B. Black Cohosh, Cayenne, Hops, Lady's Slipper, Lobelia, Mistletoe, Skullcap, Valerian, Wood Betony.

_____ C. Hops, Skullcap, Valerian.

_____ D. Valerian, Anise, Lobelia, Brigham Tea, Black Walnut, Licorice, Ginger.

Arthritis	Insomnia	Sex Depressant
Convulsions	Nervous Disorders	Skin Problems
Headache	Nightmares	Smoking
Hyperactivity	Paralysis	Stress

"D" is used in extract form and is often referred to as Antispasmodic formula for nervous problems.

24. PAIN FORMULA

_____ A. Cayenne, Valerian, Wild Lettuce

Afterpain	Cramps	Pain
Arthritis	Headache	Toothache

25. POTASSIUM FORMULAS

_____ A. Dulse, Horseradish, Horsetail, Kelp, Watercress, Wild Cabbage.

_____ B. Dulse, Horsetail, Rosemary, Sage.

Arthritis	Fatigue	Migraine Headaches
Blood Pressure	Glands	Nervous Disorders
Constipation	Heart	Obesity
Diabetes	Insomnia	Pancreas

26. POULTICE & BONE KNITTER FORMULAS

_____ A. Aloe Vera, Comfrey, Golden Seal, Slippery Elm.

_____ B. Black Walnut, Comfrey, Lobelia, Marshmallow, Mullein, Queen of the Meadow, Skullcap, White Oak Bark, Wormwood.

_____ C. Comfrey, Dandelion, Ginseng, Wood Betony.

Cuts	Infection	Poultice
Fractures	Inflammation	Skin Problems
Gout	Joints	Swelling
Hemorrhoids	Lumbago	Wounds

"A" may be taken internally or used externally. "B" is used externally. And "C" is usually used in the form of tea.

27. PROSTATE GLAND FORMULAS

_____ A. Black Cohosh, Cayenne, Ginger, Golden Seal, Gotu Kola, Kelp, Licorice, Lobelia.

_____ B. Cayenne, Ginger, Ginseng, Golden Seal, Juniper, Marshmallow, Parsley, Queen of the Meadow, Uva Ursi.

Hormones (Male)	Prostate Gland	Urinary Disorders

28. REPRODUCTIVE SYSTEM FORMULA

_____ A. Cayenne, Chickweed, Damiana, Echinacea, Garlic, Ginseng, Gotu Kola, Periwinkle, Sarsaparilla, Saw Palmetto.

Energy	Hot Flashes	Senility
Endurance	Impotence	Sex Stimulant
Frigidity	Longevity	Sterility
Hormones (Reg)	Menopause	Vitality

This combination helps to rebuild and strengthen the sex glands. It is used by both male and female. Used especially for infertility problems.

29. THROAT FORMULA

_____ A. Cinnamon, Licorice, Peppermint, Spearmint.

Bronchitis	Digestive Disorders	Laryngitis
Colds	Gas	Sore Throat
Cough	Hoarseness	Voice

This formula makes a pleasant tasting tea.

30. THYROID FORMULAS

_____ A. Cayenne, Irish Moss, Kelp, Parsley.

_____ B. Black Walnut, Iceland Moss, Irish Moss, Kelp, Parsley, Sarsaparilla, Watercress.

Energy	Goiter	Pituitary Gland
Epilepsy	Obesity	Thyroid Gland

These formulas help the Thyroid Gland produce Thyroxine which regulates either underactive or overactive Thyroid Gland. Most people who suffer from Epilepsy have an underactive Thyroid Gland.

31. ULCER & COLITIS FORMULAS

_____ A. Cayenne, Golden Seal, Myrrh.

_____ B. Comfrey, Ginger, Lobelia, Marshmallow, Slippery Elm, Wild Yam.

Canker	Gums	Thrush
Colitis	Heartburn	Ulcers
Colon	Hemorrhoids	Varicose Veins
Digestive Disorders	Mouth Sores	Wounds

32. VAGINA FORMULA

_____ A. Chickweed, Comfrey, Golden Seal, Marshmallow, Mullein, Slippery Elm, Squaw Vine, Yellow Dock.

Leucorrhea	Vagina	Yeast Infection

This formula should be used as a Bolus.

33. WEIGHT LOSS FORMULAS

_____ A. Black Walnut, Chickweed, Dandelion, Echinacea, Fennel, Gotu Kola, Hawthorn, Licorice, Mandrake, Papaya, Safflower.

_____ B. Fennel, Hawthorn, Licorice, Red Beet.

Cleansing	Constipation	Obesity

Chapter 4
HEALTH PROBLEMS

The herbs are used in capsules or teas unless otherwise indicated. The words in bold type are the ones with which we have had the most experience. See Chapter 3 for an explanation of number references for formulas.

ACNE   (See also SKIN PROBLEMS)

Aloe Vera   **Chlorophyll**   Redmond Clay
Bistort   **Dandelion**   Sarsaparilla
Burdock   Echinacea   Valerian
Cayenne   Ginseng   **White Oak Bark**
Chaparral   **Red Clover**   **Yellow Dock**
Chickweed

Formulas: #4, #9, #13
Vitamins: A, B, C, E, F, Niacin, Pyridoxine
Minerals: Potassium, Sulphur

Any of these herbs can be used internally, or as an external scrub. #4 helps to purify and cleanse the blood. #13 helps to balance the female hormones. Ginseng and Sarsaparilla help to balance the male hormones.

AFTERPAIN   (See also CHILDBIRTH)

Red Raspberry   Valerian   Wild Yam
St. Johnswort

Formulas: #5, #24

AGE SPOTS & AGING

Dandelion   Gotu Kola   Sarsaparilla
Ginseng   Licorice

Formulas: #4, #20
Vitamins: A, B, C, E
Minerals: Calcium, Selenium

ALCOHOLISM

Cayenne	Passion Flower	Skullcap
Golden Seal	Saw Palmetto	Valerian

Vitamins: A, B, C, D, E
Minerals: Magnesium

These herbs help to cleanse the system and take away the taste for alcohol.

ALLERGIES

Alfalfa	Comfrey	Lobelia
Bee Pollen	Eyebright	Marshmallow
Burdock	Fenugreek	Papaya
Chaparral	Golden Seal	Parsley
Chickweed	Juniper	

Formulas: #1, #5, #9, #12, #21
Vitamins: A, B, C, E, Pantothenic Acid
Minerals: Calcium, Magnesium, Manganese

Bee Pollen should be taken in small doses to begin with, and gradually increased to larger doses as the body builds up a resistance to the allergen.

ANEMIA

Alfalfa	Don Quai	Strawberry
Barberry	Fenugreek	Taheebo
Chlorophyll	Hops	Turkey Rhubarb
Comfrey	Kelp	**Yellow Dock**
Dandelion	St. Johnswort	

Formulas: #3, #4
Vitamins: B, C, E, Folic Acid, PABA, Pantothenic Acid
Minerals: Copper, Iron

#4 Cleanses & Purifies the blood.
Yellow Dock is very high in natural iron, and Dandelion contains the nutritive salts necessary to build good blood.

APPETITE   (To improve)

Alfalfa	Fennel	Parsley
Aloe Vera	Garlic	**Peppermint**
Barberry	Ginseng	Safflower
Blessed Thistle	Golden Seal	Strawberry
Camomile	Hops	Taheebo
Cayenne	Horseradish	Turkey Rhubarb
Dandelion	Juniper	Uva Ursi
Eucalyptus	Oat Straw	Yarrow

Formulas: #11
Vitamins: A, B, Biotin, Niacin, Thiamine
Minerals: Phosphorus, Zinc

Fennel helps normalize the appetite. Chickweed will help decrease excessive appetites when taken with #33.

ARTERIOSCLEROSIS

Cayenne	**Hawthorn**	Kelp
Garlic	Juniper	Rose Hips

Formulas: #5, #16
Vitamins: A, B, C, E, F, P, Inositol, Niacin
Minerals: Calcium, Chromium, Magnesium, Zinc

#16 helps remove cholesterol from the blood vessels.

ARTHRITIS

Alfalfa	Comfrey	Pleurisy Root
Barberry	Hawthorn	**Primrose**
Black Cohosh	Horseradish	Red Clover
Blessed Thistle	Juniper	Safflower
Brigham Tea	Licorice	Willow
Burdock	Lobelia	Yarrow
Cayenne	Oat Straw	**Yucca**
Chaparral	Parsley	

Formulas: #2, #4, #5, #23, #24, #25
Vitamins: B, C, D, E, F, P, Pantothenic Acid
Minerals: Calcium, Magnesium, Phosphorus, Potassium

Burdock reduces swelling in the joints. Yucca contains steroids and will reduce inflammation in the joints.

ASTHMA

(See also Chapter 9)

Bee Pollen
Black Cohosh
Brigham Tea
Camomile
Cayenne
Chaparral
Chickweed
Chlorophyll
Comfrey

Ginseng
Golden Seal
Horseradish
Hyssop
Licorice
Lobelia
Marshmallow
Mistletoe
Mullein

Myrrh
Nettle
Parsley
Pleurisy Root
Saw Palmetto
Slippery Elm
Thyme
Wood Betony

Formulas: #1, # 9, #21
Vitamins: A, B, B12, F, PABA, Pantothenic Acid

Honey has been used successfully. Lobelia Extract is used during an acute attack.

BAD BREATH

Alfalfa
Chlorophyll
Echinacea

Golden Seal
Irish Moss
Myrrh

Parsley
Thyme
Turkey Rhubarb

Formulas: #4, #9
Vitamins: C

Bad Breath is usually a result of congestion in the colon. Green Drinks are helpful. (See recipe in Chapter 8.) Cloves can be chewed for temporary clean breath.

BALDNESS

(Prevent Hair Loss)

Aloe Vera
Burdock
Chaparral
Horsetail

Juniper
Nettle
Sage
Watercress

White Willow
Yarrow
(Shampoo with tea)

Vitamins: B, C, E, Inositol
Minerals: Copper

The words in bold throughout the book are the ones with which we have had the most success.

61

BED WETTING

Bistort
Buchu
Corn Silk
Fennel
Hops
Horsetail

Juniper
Marshmallow
Oat Straw
Parsley
Plantain

Skullcap
St. Johnswort
Uva Ursi
Willow
Wood Betony

Formulas: #5, #19
Vitamins: A
Minerals: Magnesium

One cup of Parsley tea taken one hour before bedtime is beneficial.

BLADDER

(See KIDNEYS, see also URINARY DISORDERS)

BLEEDING

(See HEMORRHAGE, WOUNDS, Chapter 9)

BLOOD PRESSURE

(High)

Barberry
Black Cohosh
Blue Cohosh
Cayenne
Don Quai

Garlic
Ginseng
Gotu Kola
Hawthorn
Mistletoe

Passion Flower
Primrose
Skullcap
Valerian

Formulas: #16, #25
Vitamins: B, C, E, P
Minerals: Magnesium, Potassium

For Low Blood Pressure, Brigham Tea, **Dandelion,** or Parsley can be used. Cayenne, Garlic, Ginseng, Hawthorn, and Hyssop are used to regulate the Blood Pressure.

BLOOD PURIFIER

Alfalfa
Barberry
Black Cohosh
Blue Cohosh
Brigham Tea
Burdock
Camomile
Chaparral
Chlorophyll

Comfrey
Couch Grass
Dandelion
Don Quai
Echinacea
Hyssop
Licorice
Myrrh

Red Clover
Sarsaparilla
Spikenard
Strawberry
Taheebo
Yarrow
Yellow Dock
Yucca

Formulas: #3, #4
Minerals: Iron

BOILS

Barberry
Black Walnut
Burdock
Chaparral
Chickweed
Comfrey
Dandelion
Echinacea
Juniper
Lobelia
Mullein
Myrrh
Oat Straw
Red Clover
Sarsaparilla
Slippery Elm
Yellow Dock

Formulas: #4

Lobelia and Mullein are excellent as a poultice. Use 3 parts Mullein to 1 part Lobelia. The other herbs can be taken internally.

BREASTS (See FEMALE PROBLEMS)

BRONCHITIS

Black Cohosh
Camomile
Catnip
Cayenne
Chickweed
Comfrey
Couch Grass
Dandelion
Eucalyptus
Fennel
Fenugreek
Garlic
Ginger
Golden Seal
Juniper
Licorice
Lobelia
Mullein
Peppermint
Pleurisy Root
Primrose
Red Clover
Red Raspberry
Safflower
Sage
Saw Palmetto
Slippery Elm
Thyme
Uva Ursi
Wood Betony

Formulas: #8, #9, #15, #21, #29
Vitamins: A, B12, C, E

Cayenne taken with Ginger cleans out the bronchial tubes.

BRUISES (See also INFLAMMATION)

Comfrey
Don Quai
Fenugreek
Hyssop
Lobelia
Mullein
Parsley
Rose Hips
St. Johnswort
White Oak Bark
Yarrow

Formulas: #5
Vitamins: C, K, P
Minerals: Calcium

All of the above herbs are good taken internally and also applied as a poultice.

BURNS

(See also Chapter 9)

Aloe Vera	Golden Seal	**Plantain**
Burdock	Hyssop	Slippery Elm
Chickweed	Marshmallow	St. Johnswort
Comfrey	Pennyroyal	Willow

Vitamins: C, E, PABA
Minerals: Zinc

Apply ice water and keep cloths wet and cold. For shock, Cayenne may be taken. Vitamin E can be applied directly on the burn. Aloe Vera is very good for burns. It may be used internally and externally. Some Aloe Vera preparations contain lanolin which will intensify burns. Use a preparation without lanolin. Aloe Vera is especially good for acid burns.

BURSITIS

(See also ARTHRITIS, RHEUMATISM)

Alfalfa	Kelp	Willow
Burdock	Lobelia	Yarrow
Chaparral	Mullein	Yucca
Comfrey	Oat Straw	

Formulas: #2, #5
Vitamins: C, P
Minerals: Calcium, Chlorine

Mullein is often used as a poultice to give relief externally.

CANCER

(See also TUMORS, Chapter 9)

Chaparral	Ginseng	**Red Clover**
Chickweed	Golden Seal	Slippery Elm
Dandelion	Irish Moss	**Taheebo**
Eucalyptus	Parsley	Yellow Dock
Garlic	Poke Weed	

Formulas: #4, #7
Vitamins: A, B, C, E
Minerals: Magnesium, Selenium

Magnesium helps prevent cancer.

CANKER

(See MOUTH SORES)

CHILDBIRTH

(See also AFTERPAIN, LACTATION, and Chapter 5)

Blue Cohosh
Corn Silk
Kelp

Myrrh
Nutmeg
Pennyroyal

Red Raspberry
Spikenard
Squaw Vine

Formulas: #3, #5, #6
Vitamins: C, D, E
Minerals: Calcium

Nutmeg contains the alkaloid erganovine which helps the uterus contract to stop bleeding. Myrrh can be applied to the navel after the cord is removed to prevent infection.

CHILDHOOD DISEASES

(Including CHICKEN POX, MEASLES, MUMPS, RHEUMATIC FEVER, SCARLET FEVER)

Bayberry
Brigham Tea
Burdock
Camomile
Catnip
Cayenne
Garlic

Ginger
Hyssop
Lobelia
Mullein
Peppermint
Pleurisy Root
Red Clover

Red Raspberry
Rose Hips
Safflower
Skullcap
Thyme
Yarrow
Yellow Dock

Formulas: #4, #8, #18
Vitamins: A, B, C, E

Catnip or Garlic enemas are very helpful. Ginger baths are helpful. Valerian can be used for restlessness. Lobelia and Pleurisy Root are especially good for Rheumatic Fever. For itching rashes bathe the affected area in a tea made from Burdock, Golden Seal, and Yellow Dock. Mullein and Skullcap are specific for Mumps.

CIRCULATION

Bayberry
Black Cohosh
Cayenne
Chickweed

Garlic
Golden Seal
Hawthorn
Horseradish

Hyssop
Pleurisy Root
Rose Hips

Formula: #16
Vitamins: A, C, E, Lecithin, Niacin
Minerals: Calcium, Magnesium, Potassium.

Bayberry will improve the circulation. Cayenne increases the pulse rate while Black Cohosh slows it down.

CLEANSING

(See also Chapter 8)

Burdock	**Chlorophyll**	**Red Clover**
Chaparral	**Dandelion**	Taheebo
Chickweed	Lobelia	Yellow Dock

Formulas: #4, #7, #9, #20, #33
Minerals: Chlorine

Sometimes after heavy cleansing, the mucous lining in the bowel gets depleted and it is painful. Take 1/2 cup distilled water, 1 Tablespoon cider vinegar, 1 teaspoon honey and 1/4 teaspoon cayenne. Sip this several times a day to help rebuild the mucous lining and heal the colon.

COLD SORES

(See MOUTH SORES)

COLDS

(See also COUGH, FLU, FEVER, MUCOUS)

Bayberry	**Garlic**	Red Raspberry
Brigham Tea	Ginger	**Rose Hips**
Camomile	Ginseng	Sarsaparilla
Catnip	**Golden Seal**	Saw Palmetto
Cayenne	Licorice	Valerian
Comfrey	Pennyroyal	Yarrow
Fenugreek	Peppermint	

Formulas: #5, #8, #9, #14, #18, #29
Vitamins: A, B, C, E, F, P
Minerals: Calcium

COLIC

(See Chapter 5)

Blue Cohosh	**Fennel**	Valerian
Camomile	Pennyroyal	Wild Yam
Catnip	Peppermint	Yarrow

Formula: #11

COLITIS

(See also COLON)

Cayenne	Ginger	Papaya
Camomile	Golden Seal	Peppermint
Comfrey	Kelp	**Psyllium**
Fenugreek	Mandrake	**Slippery Elm**
Garlic	**Myrrh**	Turkey Rhubarb

Formulas: #5, #9, #31
Vitamins: B, E, K
Minerals: Calcium, Magnesium

COLON

Alfalfa	Chickweed	Myrrh
Aloe Vera	Comfrey	**Psyllium**
Barberry	Eucalyptus	**Slippery Elm**
Bayberry	Fenugreek	Strawberry
Camomile	Ginger	Taheebo
Chlorophyll	Hyssop	Turkey Rhubarb
Cascara Sagrada	Mullein	Yarrow

Formulas: #4, #7, #9, #31
Vitamin: B

Cascara Sagrada will improve bowel tone and bring about a premanent beneficial effect. Fenugreek helps to lubricate the colon. Hyssop and Mullein are good for decreasing mucous. To help heal the colon use 1/2 cup distilled water, 1 Tablespoon cider vinegar, 1 teaspoon honey and 1/4 teaspoon cayenne several times a day.

CONSTIPATION   (See also COLITIS, COLON)

Aloe Vera	Couch Grass	Mullein
Barberry	Dandelion	Poke Weed
Blessed Thistle	Ginseng	Psyllium
Buckthorn	Golden Seal	Red Raspberry
Cascara Sagrada	Licorice	Slippery Elm
Chickweed	Mandrake	Turkey Rhubarb

Formulas: #4, #7, #9, #25, #33
Minerals: Potassium

Aloe Vera is used internally 1 oz. 4 to 5 times a day. It is especially good for chronic constipation in older people.

CONVULSIONS & EPILEPSY

Black Cohosh	Hyssop	Pennyroyal
Blue Cohosh	Horsetail	Primrose
Catnip	Irish Moss	Skullcap
Cayenne	**Lobelia**	**Valerian**
Don Quai	**Mistletoe**	Willow
Fennel	**Passion Flower**	Wood Betony
Ginseng		

Formulas: #5, #23, #30
Vitamins: A, B, C, D, E, Pyridoxine
Minerals: Calcium, Magnesium, Silicon, Zinc

COUGH

(See also Chapter 9)

Black Cohosh	Hops	Myrrh
Cascara Sagrada	Horseradish	Parsley
Cayenne	Hyssop	Peppermint
Comfrey	Irish Moss	Pleurisy Root
Eucalyptus	Juniper	Sarasparilla
Fennel	**Licorice**	Slippery Elm
Fenugreek	**Lobelia**	St. Johnswort
Ginger	Marshmallow	Thyme
Ginseng	Mullein	Wood Betony

Formulas: #15, #21, #29
Vitamins: A, C

Ginseng, Mullein and Thyme are good for Whooping Cough.

CRAMPS

(See Also MENSTRUATION)

Muscle Cramps:

Alfalfa	**Comfrey**	Pennyroyal
Blue Cohosh	Dandelion	Peppermint
Cayenne	Don Quai	Safflower
Chaparral	Kelp	Thyme

Formulas: #3, #5
Vitamins: D, F
Minerals: Calcium

Stomach Cramps:

Blessed Thistle	Fennel	**Peppermint**
Camomile	Garlic	Slippery Elm
Cayenne	Ginger	Thyme
Cloves		

Formulas: #11, #14
Vitamins: B, E, D
Minerals: Calcium, Magnesium

The single herbs used as a tea seem to give the best results

CROUP

(See also CHILDHOOD DISEASES, Chapter 9)

Cascara Sagrada	Garlic	Mullein
Catnip	Ginger	Turkey Rhubarb
Eucalyptus	**Lobelia**	

Formula: #9

Lobelia Extract is good for acute attacks. Ginger baths are beneficial. Use Eucalyptus Oil in a steamer. Use Catnip in an enema. Lemon Juice and honey help. A cold cloth on the throat will help the swelling.

CUTS

(See WOUNDS)

DANDRUFF

Camomile	Nettle	Willow
Chaparral	**Sage**	Yarrow

Vitamins: B

Chaparral and Yarrow can be used both as a tea on the head as well as taken internally.

DIABETES AND PANCREAS

Alfalfa	Dandelion	Marshmallow
Black Cohosh	Eyebright	Oat Straw
Blueberries	False Unicorn	Queen of the Meadow
Blue Cohosh	Fenugreek	Red Raspberry
Buchu	**Golden Seal**	Saw Palmetto
Cascara Sagrada	Horseradish	Taheebo
Cayenne	Horsetail	**Uva Ursi**
Chickweed	**Juniper**	Wintergreen
Chlorophyll	Kelp	Yarrow
Comfrey	Licorice	Yellow Dock

Formulas: #3, #4, #10, #12, #20, #25
Vitamins: A, B, C, E, P, Choline, Inositol
Minerals: Potassium

Buchu is good in the first stages of Diabetes. Eyebright and #12 are used as an eyewash as well as taken internally.

DIAPER RASH
(See also SKIN PROBLEMS, Chapter 5)

Garlic	Mullein	Slippery Elm

Blend the leaf of Mullein with Vitamin E and apply to the affected area. Slippery Elm may be used internally or as a paste externally. Garlic enema may be given. Apply Garlic water to the affected area.

DIARRHEA
(See also Chapter 9)

Barberry	Ginger	**Red Raspberry**
Bayberry	Hyssop	Sage
Bistort	Marshmallow	**Slippery Elm**
Black Cohosh	Mullein	St. Johnswort
Black Walnut	**Nettle**	Thyme
Catnip	**Nutmeg**	White Oak Bark
Cloves	Peppermint	Wood Betony
Comfrey	Periwinkle	Yarrow
Garlic	Plantain	

Vitamins: B, C, Niacin
Minerals: Magnesium, Potassium

Take 1/2 teaspoon Nutmeg several times a day. Red Raspberry and Slippery Elm may be used in an enema as well as taken internally—1 Tablespoon Slippery Elm to one bag of water. Red Raspberry is used as a tea. The water from cooked rice or oatmeal may be taken orally. Slippery Elm can be added to scalded skim milk. Use 1 Tablespoon to 1 pint milk. Steep 1/2 teaspoon cloves to 1 quart of water. Take for cramping.

DIGESTIVE DISORDERS & STOMACH PROBLEMS

(See also ULCERS)

Alfalfa
Aloe Vera
Barberry
Bayberry
Blessed Thistle
Camomile
Cascara Sagrada
Catnip
Cayenne
Chlorophyll
Comfrey
Dandelion
Eyebright
False Unicorn
Fennel

Fenugreek
Garlic
Ginger
Ginseng
Golden Seal
Hops
Horseradish
Hyssop
Lobelia
Myrrh
Oat Straw
Papaya
Parsley
Peppermint
Red Raspberry

Safflower
Sage
Sarsaparilla
Skullcap
Slippery Elm
Strawberry
Taheebo
Thyme
Uva Ursi
Valerian
White Oak Bark
Wintergreen
Wood Betony
Yellow Dock

Formulas: #11, #14, #15, #29, #31
Vitamins: A, B, Biotin, Niacin
Minerals: Chlorine, Copper, Iodine, Phosphorus, Potassium, Zinc.

Digestive enzymes are helpful. Warm Peppermint tea, Cayenne, Papaya or Aloe Vera can be taken with meals.

DIZZINESS

(See also Chapter 8)

Camomile
Catnip

Peppermint
Sage

Wood Betony

Vitamin: Pyridoxine
Minerals: Potassium

DRUG WITHDRAWAL

Camomile

Ginseng

Licorice

Formulas: #22
Vitamins: B, C, E

These herbs taken together have helped those who have wanted to get off drugs.

EARACHE & EAR INFECTION

(See also Chapter 9)

Aloe Vera	Horsetail	**Mullein**
Camomile	Hyssop	Yarrow
Hops	**Lobelia**	Yellow Dock

Formulas: #8, #9, #18
Vitamins: A, C, E, Riboflavin

Yarrow and Yellow Dock can be used as teas for running ears. Place it in the ears. Baked onion poultice is placed on the ears for relief. Lobelia extract will help relieve pain. Ice bags help to disperse the blood away from the infected area and will relieve the pain.

ECZEMA

(See SKIN PROBLEMS)

ENDURANCE, ENERGY, FATIGUE & VITALITY

Alfalfa	**Dandelion**	**Hawthorn**
Bee Pollen	Don Quai	**Licorice**
Burdock	Fennel	Safflower
Cayenne	Ginger	Strawberry
Chlorophyll	**Ginseng**	Yellow Dock
Comfrey	Gotu Kola	

Formulas: #3, #16, #17, #22, #25, #28, #30
Vitamins: B, B12, E, D, F, Biotin, Riboflavin, PABA, Thiamine
Minerals: Iodine, Iron, Potassium, Zinc

Gotu Kola is especially good for mental fatigue. Safflower is used by those who suffer from Hypoglycemia to relieve muscle aches and cramps when exercising.

EPILEPSY

(See CONVULSIONS)

EYES, CATARACTS, GLAUCOMA, VISION

Bayberry	Horsetail	**Red Raspberry**
Camomile	Hyssop	Sarsaparilla
Cayenne	Marshmallow	Slippery Elm
Chaparral	Mullein	Squaw Vine
Eyebright	Oat Straw	Willow
Fennel	Parsley	Witch Hazel
Fenugreek	Plantain	Yellow Dock
Golden Seal		

Formula: #12
Vitamins: A, B, D, Inositol, Riboflavin

#12 is used by steeping 1 capsule in 1/4 cup boiling water and straining through a paper towel, then used to drop in the eyes. Hyssop packs help black eyes.

FEET

Camomile   Chlorophyll   Horsetail

Camomile is good for callouses and corns. Horsetail tea or Chlorophyll helps foot odors and foot perspiration.

FEMALE PROBLEMS   (See also AFTERPAIN, CHILDBIRTH, HEMORRHAGE, HORMONE REGULATION, LACTATION, MENOPAUSE, MENSTRUATION, MISCARRIAGE, NAUSEA, STERILITY, UTERINE PROBLEMS, VAGINAL DISORDERS, YEAST INFECTION, Chapter 5)

Black Cohosh	False Unicorn	Red Raspberry
Blessed Thistle	Ginger	Squaw Vine
Blue Cohosh	Licorice	St. Johnswort
Damiana	Marshmallow	Yarrow
Don Quai	Poke Weed	

Formulas: #13, #28
Vitamins: A

The above herbs are good for the whole female system. Poke Weed poultices will help lumps in the breast or caked breasts. Saw Palmetto will help increase breast size.

FEVER   (See also Chapter 9)

Barberry	Ginseng	Sage
Bayberry	Hops	Sarsaparilla
Blessed Thistle	Lobelia	Strawberry
Brigham Tea	Mandrake	Thyme
Catnip	Mullein	Valerian
Dandelion	Parsley	White Oak Bark
Echinacea	Passion Flower	Willow
Eucalyptus	Peppermint	Wintergreen
Fenugreek	**Rose Hips**	Yarrow
Garlic	Safflower	Yellow Dock

Formulas: #9, #14, #15, #18
Vitamins: C

Catnip tea enemas are very beneficial in lowering fevers.

73

FINGERNAILS & HAIR

Camomile	Oat Straw	Sage
Horsetail		

Formulas: #5, #25
Vitamins: A, B, F
Minerals: Calcium, Iron, Silicon, Sulphur

Horsetail helps strengthen Fingernails because of the high silicon content that is necessary for calcium absorption.
Sage and Camomile can be used to rinse the Hair.

FLU   (See also Chapter 9)

Alfalfa	**Golden Seal**	Rose Hips
Catnip	Marshmallow	Sage
Cayenne	**Peppermint**	Slippery Elm
Dandelion	Pleurisy Root	Thyme
Fenugreek	Red Clover	**Yarrow**
Ginger	**Red Raspberry**	Yellow Dock

Formulas: #5, #8, #15, #18
Vitamins: A, C, E, P
Minerals: Calcium

#14 is good for Intestinal Flu and Vomiting. Catnip and Peppermint are good used together at the onset of the flu.

FRACTURES

Alfalfa	Dandelion	Plantain
Aloe Vera	**Horsetail**	Red Raspberry
Cayenne	Irish Moss	**Slippery Elm**
Chlorophyll	Kelp	Yarrow
Comfrey	Parsley	Yellow Dock

Formulas: #5, #26
Vitamins: D
Minerals: Calcium, Magnesium, Phosphorus

Slippery Elm and #26 can be used as a poultice over the Fracture.

The words in bold throughout the book are the ones with which we have had the most success.

GALL BLADDER AND
GALL STONES   (See also Chapter 9)

Barberry	Fennel	Peppermint
Blessed Thistle	Garlic	Primrose
Buckthorn	Golden Seal	Safflower
Burdock	Hyssop	Strawberry
Cascara Sagrada	Mandrake	White Oak Bark
Comfrey	Mistletoe	Willow
Couch Grass	Oat Straw	Wormwood
Dandelion	Parsley	Yellow Dock

Formulas: #20
Vitamins: A, B, C, D, E, Inositol
Minerals: Magnesium, Sulphur

GAS   (See also DIGESTIVE DISORDERS)

Barberry	**Ginger**	Sage
Blessed Thistle	Ginseng	Spearmint
Camomile	Hyssop	Thyme
Catnip	Juniper	Valerian
Cayenne	Papaya	Wild Yam
Fennel	**Peppermint**	Willow
Garlic	Safflower	Wormwood

Formulas: #11, #29
Vitamins: B, Thiamine

Hydrochloric acid is sometimes helpful. Digestive enzymes can be used. Ginseng and Horseradish are used specifically for colon gas.

GLANDS   (See LYMPH)

GOUT   (See also ARTHRITIS, RHEUMATISM)

Alfalfa	Fennel	**Safflower**
Buckthorn	Horseradish	Sarsaparilla
Burdock	Oat Straw	St. Johnswort
Comfrey	Parsley	Willow
Corn Silk	Pennyroyal	Wood Betony
Couch Grass	**Primrose**	Yellow Dock
Dandelion	Queen of the Meadow	Yucca

Formulas: #2, #5, #26
Vitamins: B, C, E
Minerals: Calcium, Magnesium, Potassium

Gout is caused by excessive Uric Acid. Primrose and Safflower will help eliminate Uric Acid buildup.

HALITOSIS   (See BAD BREATH)

HAYFEVER

Alfalfa	Chaparral	**Juniper**
Bayberry	Chickweed	Lobelia
Bee Pollen	Comfrey	Marshmallow
Brigham Tea	Eyebright	Mullein
Burdock	Fenugreek	Parsley
Cayenne	Golden Seal	

Formulas: #1, #12, #21
Vitamins: A, C, E

HEADACHE   (See also MIGRAINE HEADACHE)

Black Cohosh	**Ginger**	Skullcap
Blessed Thistle	Hops	**Thyme**
Brigham Tea	Lobelia	Turkey Rhubarb
Camomile	**Passion Flower**	Willow
Catnip	Pennyroyal	Wintergreen
Comfrey	Peppermint	**Wood Betony**
Fenugreek	Sage	Yarrow

Formulas: #5, #15, #23, #24
Vitamins: B
Minerals: Calcium, Potassium

Black Cohosh is especially good for pains in the back of the head.

HEART

Barberry	**Hawthorn**	Safflower
Black Cohosh	Horsetail	St. Johnswort
Blue Cohosh	Lobelia	Valerian
Cayenne	Mistletoe	Wintergreen
Chlorophyll	Oat Straw	Wood Betony
Garlic	Rose Hips	

Formulas: #16, #25
Vitamins: A, B, C, D, E, Lecithin, Thiamine, Biotin, Inositol
Minerals: Calcium, Iodine, Iron, Magnesium, Potassium

Barberry in low doses acts as a heart stimulant, in high doses it will slow down the heart rate. Hawthorn is used to strengthen the heart. Sherpherd's Purse normalizes heart action. Lobelia helps heart palpitations. Mineral water taken internally is also good for the heart.

HEARTBURN   (See DIGESTIVE DISORDERS)

HEMORRHAGE

External:
Bistort
Camomile
Cayenne
Comfrey
Dandelion
Echinacea

Eyebright
Golden Seal
Horsetail
Plaintain
Red Raspberry
Sage

Slippery Elm
St. Johnswort
White Oak Bark
Witch Hazel
Willow

Internal:
Bayberry
Bistort
Cayenne
Chickweed
Comfrey

Ginseng
Golden Seal
Mullein
Plantain

St. Johnswort
White Oak Bark
Willow
Yarrow

Lungs:
Bayberry
Cayenne

Chickweed
Ginger

Mullein
Yarrow

Nosebleed:
Brigham Tea
Golden Seal

Horsetail
Mullein

White Oak Bark
Witch Hazel

Urinary:
Comfrey
Marshmallow

Nettle

White Oak Bark

Uterus & Vagina:
Bayberry
Bistort
Corn Silk

False Unicorn
Golden Seal
Mistletoe

White Oak Bark
Witch Hazel

Vitamin: K

Bistort, Golden Seal, and White Oak Bark tea can be used as a douche, enema or snuffed up the nose. Yarrow is taken internally to reduce the clotting time. Chlorophyll helps the blood to clot as it is rich in Vitamin K. Marshmallow can be used for bladder hemorrhage by simmering 1 oz. of Marshmallow in 2 cups of milk and drinking 1/2 cup each 1/2 hour. For Bowel hemorrhage use 1 oz. Mullein to 2 cups of milk simmered slowly and drink 2 cups every bowel movement. Lemon juice diluted and taken cold is also good for internal hemorrhage. Taheebo is used for all types of hemorrhage.

HEMORRHOIDS & PILES   (See also Chapter 9)

Aloe Vera	Chlorophyll	**Slipper Elm**
Buckthorn	Golden Seal	Taheebo
Burdock	Mullein	Turkey Rhubarb
Camomile	Plantain	Uva Ursi
Cascara Sagrada	Poke Weed	**White Oak Bark**
Cayenne	**Psyllium**	**Witch Hazel**
Chickweed	Safflower	Yarrow

Formulas: #26, #31
Vitamins: A, B, C, E, Lecithin
Minerals: Potassium

Golden Seal and White Oak Bark packs help to reduce swelling and alleviate pain. Put Vitamin E on a piece of peeled, raw potato the size of a little finger and insert it at night to reduce swelling and pain of hemorrhoids.

HEPATITIS   (See LIVER)

HIGH BLOOD PRESSURE   (See BLOOD PRESSURE)

HOARSENESS

Bayberry	Hops	Marshmallow
Chickweed	Horseradish	Mullein
Comfrey	Horsetail	Plantain
Fennel	Hyssop	Sage
Fenugreek	**Licorice**	Slippery Elm
Golden Seal	Lobelia	

Formulas: #21, #29
Vitamins: C, E

Any of the above herbs are good as a gargle or tea.

HORMONE REGULATION

Female:
Black Cohosh	**Damiana**	Sarsaparilla
Blessed Thistle	**Don Quai**	Saw Palmetto

Formulas: #6, #28

Male:
Ginseng	**Sarsaparilla**

Formulas: #27, #28
Minerals: Chlorine, Potassium

Ginseng and Sarsaparilla taken together are very helpful in balancing the male hormones.

HYPOGLYCEMIA

Alfalfa	**Dandelion**	**Licorice**
Bee Pollen	Don Quai	Lobelia
Black Cohosh	Hawthorn	Marshmallow
Blue Cohosh	Horseradish	**Safflower**
Catnip	**Juniper**	Skullcap
Chlorophyll	Kelp	Valerian

Formulas: #5, #10, #17
Vitamins: B, C, E, Pantothenic Acid
Minerals: Magnesium, Potassium

Some people who have Hypoglycemia cannot handle Golden Seal as it tends to lower the blood sugar. Safflower is good to take before exercise.

IMPOTENCE   (See STERILITY)

INDIGESTION   (See DIGESTIVE DISORDERS)

INFECTION

Cayenne	**Garlic**	Myrrh
Comfrey	**Golden Seal**	Poke Weed
Echinacea		

Formulas: #4, #18, #26
Vitamins: A, C, E, P

#26 is used as a poultice on external injuries to help prevent infection or to draw it out. Golden Seal and Garlic both act as antibiotics. Cayenne and Garlic are used as a douche for vaginal infection.

INFLAMMATION & SWELLING

(See also BRUISES)

Camomile
Chickweed
Comfrey
Ginseng
Golden Seal

Hyssop
Marshmallow
Poke Weed
Rose Hips
Slippery Elm

Wintergreen
Witch Hazel
Wood Betony
Yellow Dock
Yucca

Formulas: #2, #4, #26
Vitamins: A, C, E, F

Comfrey and Wood Betony are good for sprains. Onion packs are also good. Yucca contains steroids that help eliminate inflammation in the joints.

INSECT BITES & BEE STINGS

Bistort
Black Cohosh
Comfrey
Echinacea
Fennel
Garlic

Hyssop
Juniper
Lobelia
Nettle
Parsley
Plantain

Rose Hips
Sage
Skullcap
St. Johnswort
Wood Betony

Formulas: #1, #4,
Vitamins: C
Minerals: Calcium, Magnesium

Redmond Clay can be used externally to draw out the stinger.

INSOMNIA

Catnip
Chaparral
Dandelion
Don Quai
Hawthorn
Hops

Lobelia
Mullein
Passion Flower
Peach
Peppermint
Primrose

Red Clover ·
Skullcap
Squaw Vine
Taheebo
Valerian
Yarrow

Formulas: #5, #23
Vitamins: B, D, Thiamine, Pyridoxine, Niacin
Minerals: Calcium, Iron, Potassium

ITCHING

(See also ECZEMA, SKIN PROBLEMS)

Buckthorn
Burdock
Chickweed

Golden Seal
Pennyroyal
Peppermint

Plantain
Yellow Dock

Formula: #4
Vitamins: B

Peppermint tea bath is very soothing. Yellow Dock can be taken internally to alleviate itching almost anywhere in the body.

KIDNEYS, BLADDER, & STONES

(See also HEMORRHAGE Chapter 9)

Alfalfa
Barberry
Black Cohosh
Blessed Thistle
Blue Cohosh
Brigham Tea
Buchu
Burdock
Camomile
Catnip
Cayenne
Chaparral
Comfrey
Corn Silk

Couch Grass
Cramp Bark
Dandelion
Echinacea
Golden Seal
Hawthorn
Horseradish
Horsetail
Hyssop
Juniper
Kelp
Marshmallow
Nettle
Oat Straw

Parsley
Peach
Plantain
Queen of the Meadow
Rose Hips
Saw Palmetto
Slippery Elm
Taheebo
Thyme
Uva Ursi
White Oak Bark
Wood Betony
Yarrow
Yellow Dock

Formulas: #19
Vitamins: A, B, C, E, F, Choline, Pantothenic Acid
Minerals: Magnesium, Potassium

Lemon Juice helps take the edge off Kidney Stones. #19 and Thyme help dissolve Kidney Stones. Marshmallow is used for Bladder Hemorrhage. (See Hemorrhage)

LACTATION

Alfalfa
Blessed Thistle

Chlorophyll
Fennel

Marshmallow
Red Raspberry

Formulas: #5
Vitamins: A, D, Choline
Minerals: Calcium, Iodine, Manganese, Phosphorus

The above herbs will promote and enrich the milk flow. Papaya may be added to cow's milk to resemble breast milk and make it more digestible. To dry up or decrease the milk flow, use Black Walnut Bark, Parsley or Sage.

LARYNGITIS (See HOARSENESS)

LEUCORRHEA (See VAGINAL DISORDERS)

LIVER, JAUNDICE & HEPATITIS

Aloe Vera
Barberry
Black Cohosh
Blessed Thistle
Buckthorn
Burdock
Camomile
Cascara Sagrada
Cayenne
Chlorophyll
Couch Grass
Dandelion
False Unicorn

Fennel
Garlic
Golden Seal
Hops
Horseradish
Horsetail
Hyssop
Irish Moss
Lobelia
Mandrake
Oat Straw
Papaya
Parsley

Peppermint
Poke Weed
Rose Hips
Safflower
Strawberry
Thyme
Turkey Rhubarb
Uva Ursi
White Oak Bark
Wood Betony
Wormwood
Yellow Dock

Formulas: #4, #20
Vitamins: A, B, C, E, Choline, Folic Acid. Pantothenic Acid
Minerals: Copper, Sulphur

LONGEVITY (See also ENDURANCE,

Bee Pollen
Damiana
Don Quai

False Unicorn
Ginseng
Gotu Kola

Licorice
Sarsaparilla

Formulas: #28
Vitamins: A, B, C, E, Riboflavin, Pantothenic Acid
Minerals: Calcium

LOW BLOOD PRESSURE (See BLOOD PRESSURE)

The words in bold throughout the book are the ones with which we have had the most success.

LUMBAGO

(Lower Back Pain. See also CRAMPS: Leg and muscle)

Bayberry
Black Cohosh
Comfrey
Juniper

Oat Straw
Parsley
Plantain
Poke Weed

Queen of the Meadow
Slippery Elm
Uva Ursi
Valerian

Formulas: #5, #26
Vitamins: B, E, Thiamine
Minerals: Calcium

LUNGS, EMPHYSEMA, PLEURISY & PNEUMONIA

Bayberry
Black Cohosh
Blessed Thistle
Burdock
Cayenne
Chickweed
Comfrey
Eucalyptus
Fenugreek
Garlic
Ginger

Ginseng
Horseradish
Horsetail
Hyssop
Irish Moss
Lobelia
Licorice
Marshmallow
Mullein
Myrrh
Oat Straw

Pennyroyal
Plantain
Pleurisy Root
Rose Hips
Sage
Slippery Elm
St. Johnswort
Thyme
Yarrow

Formulas: #18, #21
Vitamins: A, C, E

For Pleurisy use 1/2 teaspoon Cayenne, 1 Tablespoon Lobelia, and 3 Tablespoons Slippery Elm. Mix with mineral water. Use as a pack to the chest for only 1 hour. Fennel, Garlic and Rose Hips are especially good for Emphysema. Also Fenugreek and Comfrey used together are good for Emphysema.

MILD MUSTARD PLASTER:

May be left over night. Also used for Babies. 1 T. Ginger, 1 T. dry mustard, 1 T. turpentine, 1 T. salt, 3 T. lard or shortening.

MUSTARD PLASTER:

1 T. Mustard, 3 T. flour, mix with water and leave until skin is pink. 1 egg may be added to prevent blisters.

LYMPH & SWOLLEN GLANDS

Burdock	Lobelia	Poke Weed
Cayenne	Mullein	Saw Palmetto
Echinacea	Myrrh	Yarrow
Golden Seal	Nettle	Yellow Dock

Formulas: #4, #14, #18
Vitamins: A, C, E, Pantothenic Acid

Exercise is probably one of the most important things that can be done to help lymph move through the body. Saw Palmetto helps to strengthen the glands.

MENOPAUSE & HOT FLASHES

Black Cohosh	Ginseng	Licorice
Blue Cohosh	Gotu Kola	**Passion Flower**
Damiana	Hawthorn	Sarsaparilla
Don Quai	Kelp	Valerian

Formulas: #13, #28
Vitamins: A, B, C, D, E
Minerals: Calcium

Black Cohosh and Ginseng will supply a natural estrogen. Damiana, Don Quai, Passion Flower and Sarsaparilla are especially good for Hot Flashes.

MENSTRUATION

Cramps and Difficulties:

Black Cohosh	Don Quai	Pennyroyal
Blessed Thistle	False Unicorn	Peppermint
Blue Cohosh	Ginger	Red Raspberry
Catnip	Hops	Strawberry
Chlorophyll	Myrrh	Wild Yam
Cramp Bark	Parsley	Yarrow

To Decrease excessive flow:

Bayberry	Golden Seal	Red Raspberry
Bistort	Marshmallow	Uva Ursi
Cayenne	**Mistletoe**	White Oak Bark
Comfrey	Plantain	Wood Betony
False Unicorn		

Promote Supressed Menstruation:

Black Cohosh   Ginger   Sage
Blue Cohosh   Ginseng   Skullcap
Brigham Tea   Horsetail   Squaw Vine
Camomile   Parsley   St. Johnswort
Catnip   Pennyroyal   Valerian
Cramp Bark   Safflower   Wild Yam
Fennel

Formulas: #13, #24
Vitamins: B, C, E
Minerals: Iodine

#13 and #24 are used for cramps
Most of the herbs used to promote menstruation contain steroids which may affect the hormone regulation of the body. See Chapter 5.

MIGRAINE HEADACHES   (See also HEADACHES)

Blessed Thistle   **Fenugreek**   Peppermint
Camomile   Garlic   **Thyme**
Cayenne   Hops   Valerian
Eucalyptus   **Lobelia**   **Wood Betony**
Fennel   Nutmeg

Formulas: #5, #15, #25
Vitamins: B12, F, PABA
Minerals: Calcium, Potassium

Camomile will help prevent migraine headaches. Fenugreek, Thyme, and Wood Betony are used in combination. Nutmeg contains an alkaloid, Ergotamine which constricts the blood vessels. Migraine Headaches can come from various sources—Diet, neck injuries, nerves, stress, etc.

MISCARRIAGE

Bayberry   Cramp Bark   **Lobelia**
Catnip   **False Unicorn** Wild Yam
Cayenne   Hawthorn

Vitamins: E, P

False Unicorn and Lobelia can be used together.

MOUTH SORES, CANKER, THRUSH, SORE GUMS, & PYORRHEA

Aloe Vera	Chickweed	Plantain
Barberry	Chlorophyll	Poke Weed
Bayberry	Comfrey	Sage
Bistort	Echinacea	**White Oak Bark**
Black Walnut	**Golden Seal**	Willow
Burdock	**Myrrh**	Witch Hazel
Cayenne	**Red Raspberry**	

Formulas: #4, #31
Vitamins: A, B, B12, C, E, Niacin, Riboflavin
Minerals: Iron, Magnesium, Phosphorus

Red Raspberry is good for cankers. Rinse mouth with Mineral water. Use Myrrh extract. Use White Oak Bark and Golden Seal teas to rinse the mouth and gums.

MUCOUS MEMBRANES
& MUCOUS   (See also SINUS CONGESTION)

Bayberry	Juniper	Red Raspberry
Comfrey	Licorice	Sage
Echinacea	Lobelia	Sarsaparilla
Eucalyptus	Marshmallow	**Slippery Elm**
Fennel	Mullein	**Thyme**
Fenugreek	Myrrh	Uva Ursi
Golden Seal	Papaya	Witch Hazel
Horseradish	Pennyroyal	Yarrow
Hyssop	Pleurisy Root	

Formulas: #1, #8, #18, #21
Vitamins: A, C, E

NAUSEA & MORNING SICKNESS

Alfalfa	Hops	**Red Raspberry**
Catnip	Kelp	Sage
Eucalpytus	Peach	Spearmint
Fennel	Peppermint	Wild Yam
Ginger		

Formulas: #14
Vitamins: B, C
Minerals: Calcium

There are herbal oil combinations available to help with nausea.

NERVOUS DISORDERS

Black Cohosh
Blue Cohosh
Burdock
Camomile
Cascara Sagrada
Catnip
Celery
Cramp Bark
Don Quai
Eucalpytus
Fennel
Ginger
Golden Seal
Hawthorn
Hops
Horsetail
Hyssop
Lettuce
Lobelia
Marshmallow
Mistletoe
Myrrh
Oat Straw
Passion Flower
Peach Leaves
Pennyroyal
Peppermint
Primrose
Queen of the
   Meadow
Red Clover
Red Raspberry
Sage
Skullcap
Squaw Vine
St. Johnswort
Strawberry
Taheebo
Thyme
Valerian
Wild Yam
Wood Betony
Yarrow
Yellow Dock

Formulas: #5, #23, #25
Vitamins: B, D, E, Inositol Niacin, Pyrodoxine, Riboflavin, Thiamine
Minerals: Calcium, Iodine, Iron, Magnesium, Phosphorus, Potassium,
       Silicon, Sodium.

Cayenne, Eucalpytus and Yellow Dock are especially good for Paralysis. For Shingles, apple cider vinegar may be applied externally. Use Thyme as a salve. Oil of Peppermint can be used externally as well.

NIGHTMARES

Catnip
Hops
Lobelia
Peppermint
Skullcap
Thyme

Formulas: #5, #23
Vitamins: B
Minerals: Calcium

NIGHT SWEATS

Hops
Hyssop
Nettle
Sage
Strawberry Leaves
Yarrow

Vitamins: D

NOSEBLEED   (See HEMORRHAGE)

OBESITY

Burdock	Golden Seal	Irish Moss
Chaparral	Hops	**Kelp**
Chickweed	Horsetail	Uva Ursi
Fennel		

Formulas: #5, #13, #25, #30, #33
Vitamins: B, C, E, Lecithin
Minerals: Calcium, Iodine, Potassium

#33 can be taken with Chickweed. Start slowly as the herbs will cleanse the body. If too much is taken at once diarrhea may occur. If weight loss is too slow, add more Chickweed.

PAIN   (See also AFTERPAIN, CRAMPS, HEADACHE, MIGRAINE HEADACHE)

Camomile	Peppermint	Wild Lettuce
Catnip	Poke Weed	**Wild Yam**
Corn Silk	Primrose	**Wintergreen**
Lobelia	Taheebo	Wood Betony
Marshmallow	**Valerian**	Wormwood

Formulas: #5, #24
Vitamins: C
Minerals: Calcium

Taheebo is especially good for pain associated with Cancer.

PANCREAS   (See DIABETES)

PARASITES & WORMS

Aloe Vera	Hops	**Sage**
Bistort	Horseradish	Slippery Elm
Black Walnut	Hyssop	St. Johnswort
Buckthorn	**Male Fern**	Thyme
Camomile	Onion	Valerian
Catnip	Papaya	White Oak Bark
Couch Grass	Poke Weed	Wood Betony
Garlic	**Pumpkin Seeds**	Wormwood

Formulas: #7, #9
Vitamin: Folic Acid

Black Walnut taken with #7 will kill most Parasites and Worms. Small children can eat Pumpkin Seeds and drink Camomile tea.

PERSPIRATION

To Decrease:
Wood Betony

To Promote:

Buckthorn	Hyssop	Pleurisy Root
Catnip	Pennyroyal	Safflower
Ginger	Peppermint	Yarrow

A Ginger bath will help produce perspiration and clean the pores in any type of illness, especially good for colds and flu.

Odor:
Chlorophyll   Horsetail (foot bath)

Minerals: Magnesium

PITUITARY GLAND

Alfalfa	**Gotu Kola**	Parsley
Ginseng	Kelp	Yellow Dock

Formulas: #3, #22, #30
Vitamins: C, E, Lecithin, PABA

PNEUMONIA   (See LUNGS)

POISON IVY—OAK

Aloe Vera	Lobelia	Rose Hips
Black Walnut	**Mullein**	**Yellow Dock**
Burdock	Plantain	

Formulas: #4
Vitamins: High doses of C

Within a 10 foot radius of the Poisonous plant there will be something to counteract the poison. Rub the leaf on the affected part. This should be done as soon as possible for best results. Cornstarch has been known to help stop the itching temporarily when used as a paste. Black Walnut extract and Aloe Vera gel are also used for itching. The system needs to be cleaned out by enemas.

POISONING

Blood:

Chickweed	Echinacea	Plantain

Food:

Camomile	Lobelia

Ptomaine:

Eat two heads of Iceburg Lettuce

Vitamins: A, C, E, Folic Acid

Camomile will induce vomiting without depressing the systems. It should be taken in large doses.

Lobelia will cause vomiting if taken in large doses therefore it is good when the stomach contents need to be removed as in the case of poisoning.

PREGNANCY   (See Chapter 5)

PROSTATE GLAND   (See also URINARY DISORDERS)

Bee Pollen	Garlic	Parsley
Buchu	Ginseng	Queen of the Meadow
Chaparral	Golden Seal	Saw Palmetto
Corn Silk	**Juniper**	Taheebo
Damiana	Kelp	**Uva Ursi**
Echinacea		

Formulas: #7, #27
Vitamins: A, B, C, E, F
Minerals: Zinc

Enlarged prostate may obstruct the flow of urine.

PSORIASIS   (See SKIN PROBLEMS)

RHEUMATISM

(See also ARTHRITIS, GOUT)

Alfalfa
Barberry
Black Cohosh
Brigham Tea
Buchu
Buckthorn
Burdock
Cayenne
Chaparral
Chickweed

Comfrey
Fennel
Garlic
Hawthorn
Hops
Horseradish
Lobelia
Oat Straw
Pleurisy Root
Poke Weed

Primrose
Queen of the Meadow
Red Clover
Red Raspberry
Sarsaparilla
Skullcap
Taheebo
Willow
Wintergreen
Yucca

Formulas: #2, #4, #5
Vitamins: C, E
Minerals: Calcium, Magnesium

RINGWORM

Black Walnut
Garlic
Golden Seal

Lobelia
Poke Weed
Sarsaparilla

Taheebo
White Oak Bark

Formuals: #4

Apply apple cider vinegar to the skin, or use Black Walnut extract.
Cleanse the system with Garlic enemas.

SENILITY

(See also AGE SPOTS, ENDURANCE)

Alfalfa
Damiana
Dandelion

False Unicorn
Ginseng
Gotu Kola

Licorice
Sarsaparilla
Yellow Dock

Formulas: #3, #22, #28
Vitamins: A, B, C, E

SEX DESIRE

(See also STERILITY)

Depressant:

Hops
Sage

Skullcap

Willow

Stimulant:

Damiana
Ginseng

Licorice
Safflower

Slippery Elm

Formulas: #23, #28
Vitamins: E

#23 will depress the Sex Desire while #28 will increase the Sex Desire.

SHOCK

Cayenne	Lobelia	Valerian
Ginger	Myrrh	

Formulas: #16
Vitamins: C, E

SINUS CONGESTION   (See also MUCOUS MEMBRANE)

Bayberry	Fennel	Horseradish
Brigham Tea	**Fenugreek**	Hyssop
Cayenne	Garlic	Mullein
Comfrey	Ginger	Rose Hips
Eucalyptus	Golden Seal	Witch Hazel

Formulas: #1, #9, #18, #21
Vitamins: A, C, Pantothenic Acid

Bayberry, Brigham Tea, and Golden Seal may be snuffed up the nose. Another good remedy is to boil 1 pint water and add 1 teaspoon of salt and 1 teaspoon of soda, cool and add 1 Tablespoon Witch Hazel and use this solution to snuff up the nose and spit out. Do this several times a day.

SKIN PROBLEMS   (See also ACNE, ITCHING)

Aloe Vera	Don Quai	Safflower
Barberry	Ginger Baths	Sage
Bistort	Golden Seal	Sarsaparilla
Black Cohosh	Gotu Kola	St. Johnswort
Black Walnut	Horseradish	Taheebo
Brigham Tea	Hyssop	Thyme
Buckthorn	Kelp	White Oak Bark
Burdock	Mullein	Wintergreen
Chaparral	Pennyroyal	Yarrow
Chickweed	Poke Weed	**Yellow Dock**
Comfrey	**Red Clover**	Yucca
Dandelion	**Redmond Clay**	

Formulas: #4, #5, #7, #23, #26
Vitamins: A, B, C, F, P, Biotin, Niacin, PABA, Pantothenic Acid, Pyridoxine, Riboflavin

Minerals: Iron, Silicon, Sulphur

Aloe Vera is used internally as well as externally.

SMOKING

(See also COUGH, Chapter 8)

Black Cohosh
Blue Cohosh
Catnip

Echinacea
Hops
Peppermint

Skullcap
Slippery Elm
Valerian

Formulas: #23
Vitamins: C

Hops, Skullcap, Slippery Elm, and Valerian taken together kills the desire for Tobacco.

SORE THROAT

(See also HOARSENESS, Chapter 9)

Aloe Vera
Barberry
Bayberry
Burdock
Cayenne
Chickweed
Chlorophyll
Comfrey
Eucalyptus
Fenugreek

Garlic
Golden Seal
Horehound
Hyssop
Juniper
Licorice
Marshmallow
Mullein
Myrrh
Pennyroyal

Pineapple
Red Raspberry
Rose Hips
Sage
Slippery Elm
Thyme
White Oak Bark
Witch Hazel
Yarrow

Formulas: #14, #15, #18, #29
Vitamins: A, C, E

Any of these herbs may be used as a gargle. Garlic enemas are used to fight infection. A towel wrung out of salt water and applied around the neck will help a sore throat. Place plastic over the towel to keep the pillow dry.

SPLEEN

Barberry
Camomile
Cascara Sagrada
Cayenne

Dandelion
Golden Seal
Horseradish
Parsley

Uva Ursi
Yellow Dock
Yarrow

Formulas: #4, #20
Vitamins: C, Choline

STERILITY, FRIGIDITY, & IMPOTENCE

Chickweed
Damiana
False Unicorn

Fenugreek
Ginseng
Plantain

Safflower
Sarsaparilla
Saw Palmetto

Formulas: #13, #22, #28
Vitamins: E
Minerals: Iodine

SWELLING   (See INFLAMMATION)

THRUSH   (See MOUTH SORES)

THYROID & GOITER

Black Cohosh
Chlorophyll
Irish Moss

Kelp
Parsley

Poke Weed
White Oak Bark

Formulas: #3, #30
Vitamins: C, D, E, F, Thiamine
Minerals: Chlorine, Iodine, Potassium, Zinc

Bayberry, Golden Seal, Myrrh are used for low Thyroid. Poke Weed is especially good for Goiter.

TONSILLITIS   (See also Chapter 9)

Aloe Vera
Burdock
Cayenne
Chlorophyll
Comfrey

Echinacea
Garlic
Golden Seal
Pleurisy Root
Rose Hips

Sage
Slippery Elm
White Oak Bark
Wood Betony

Formulas: #4, #18
Vitamins: A, C, E, P, Pantothenic Acid

TOOTHACHE & TEETH

Camomile	Horsetail	Myrrh
Cloves	Hyssop	Pennyroyal
Ginger	**Lobelia**	**Primrose**
Hops	Mullein	**White Oak Bark**

Formulas #5, #24
Vitamins: A, C
Minerals: Calcium, Magnesium, Phosphorus, Silicon

Brush teeth with Black Walnut powder to help remove stains. Comfrey will help decayed teeth. White Oak Bark will help set loose teeth. Primrose Oil or Oil of Cloves will help relieve Toothache.

TUMORS   (See also CANCER)

Chaparral	Mullein	**Red Clover**
Chickweed	Plantain	**Taheebo**
Lobelia	Poke Weed	Yellow Dock

Formulas: #4, #7

A poultice of 3 parts Mullein to 1 part Lobelia will help reduce the swelling.

ULCERS   (See also DIGESTIVE DISORDERS)

Alfalfa	**Golden Seal**	Sage
Bayberry	Hops	**Slippery Elm**
Bistort	Horsetail	St. Johnswort
Burdock	Hyssop	Taheebo
Cayenne	Licorice	Valerian
Chickweed	**Myrrh**	**White Oak Bark**
Chlorophyll	Pennyroyal	Wild Yam
Comfrey	Plantain	Yarrow
Eucalyptus	Poke Weed	Yellow Dock
Fenugreek	Psyllium	Yucca
Garlic	Red Raspberry	

Formulas: #5, #31
Vitamins: B, C, E
Minerals: Calcium

The words in bold throughout the book are the ones with which we have had the most success.

URINARY DISORDERS

(See also KIDNEYS, HEMORRHAGE, WATER RETENTION)

Blessed Thistle
Buchu
Corn Silk
Cramp Bark

Echinacea
Goldenrod
Horsetail
Juniper

Corn Silk
Nettle
Uva Ursi

Formulas: #10, #19, #27
Vitamins: A, C, E

UTERINE PROBLEMS

Alfalfa
Aloe Vera
Black Cohosh
Catnip
Corn Silk

Eucalyptus
False Unicorn
Golden Seal
Horsetail
Myrrh

Queen of the Meadow
Red Raspberry
Slippery Elm
Wild Yam
Yarrow

Formulas: #13
Vitamins: E

Bayberry, False Unicorn, Uva Ursi, and White Oak Bark are used for Prolapsed Uterus.

VAGINAL DISORDERS

Aloe Vera
Barberry
Bayberry
Bistort
Black Walnut
Blessed Thistle
Blue Cohosh
Comfrey
False Unicorn

Fenugreek
Garlic
Ginger
Golden Seal
Horsetail
Marshmallow
Myrrh
Nettle
Plantain

Queen of the Meadow
Red Raspberry
Slippery Elm
Thyme
Uva Ursi
White Oak Bark
Wintergreen
Witch Hazel

Formulas: #13, #32
Vitamins: A, C, E

The following can be used as a Douche either alone or in combination: Aloe Vera, Horsetail, Garlic and Cayenne. White Oak Bark can be added for more effectiveness. Mineral Water can also be used. Bistort is used for bleeding from the vagina. Marshmallow tea is used for vaginal irritation.

VARICOSE VEINS   (See also CIRCULATION)

Bayberry   **White Oak Bark**   **Witch Hazel**
Cayenne   Wintergreen   Wood Betony
Taheebo

Formulas: #5, #16, #31
Minerals: Iodine

White Oak Bark can be taken internally. Witch Hazel or White Oak
Bark tea can be used externally.

VENEREAL DISEASES

Black Walnut   Golden Seal   Wintergreen
Buchu   Taheebo   Witch Hazel
Burdock   Uva Ursi   Yellow Dock
Echinacea

Formulas: #4
Vitamins: A, B, C, E

These herbs can be taken internally and used in tea form externally
or as a douche to relieve pain and itching.

VOMITING   (See NAUSEA)

WARTS

Buckthorn   Garlic   Milkweed
Chaparral   Mandrake   Mullein

Vitamins: A, C, E

The milk from the Milkweed plant is good. Also, Vitamin E and Castor
Oil have helped in many cases.

WATER RETENTION

Blue Cohosh
Burdock
Catnip
Cornsilk
Couch Grass
Dandelion
Fennel
Fenugreek
Golden Seal

Gotu Kola
Hawthorn
Hops
Horseradish
Horsetail
Juniper
Parsley
Peach Bark
Pleurisy Root

Queen of the Meadow
Safflower
'Slippery Elm
St. Johnswort
Taheebo
Uva Ursi
Wintergreen
Yarrow

Formulas: #3, #5, #19
Vitamins: B, C
Minerals: Calcium, Potassium

WORMS   (See PARASITES)

WOUNDS AND SORES

Aloe Vera
Bayberry
Bistort
Burdock
Camomile
Cayenne
Chaparral
Chickweed
Comfrey
Dandelion

Echinacea
Golden Seal
Horseradish
Horsetail
Lobelia
Myrrh
Papaya
Peach Bark
Plantain
Sage

Slippery Elm
St. Johnswort
Taheebo
Valerian
White Oak Bark
Willow
Witch Hazel
Wood Betony
Yarrow
Yucca

Formulas: #4, #5, #26, #31
Vitamins: A, B, C, E
Minerals: Calcium

These herbs may be used internally or as poultices.

YEAST INFECTION

Cayenne   Garlic   White Oak Bark

Formulas: #32
Vitamins: A, C, E.

Fresh Garlic as a douche will usually clear up a Yeast Infection in 3 days. White Oak Bark may be added to the Garlic for better results. Fresh, Homemade yogurt can be inserted in the Vagina. For babies, Garlic Water may be used to wash the affected area.

Chapter 5

PREGNANCIES, BABIES AND NURSING

A. PREGNANCY

Proper diet is one of the most important and valuable practices during pregnancy. It should consist mostly of fresh fruits and vegetables with some whole grain cereals and nuts.

Exercise is also an important part of a successful pregnancy. Some mothers find it beneficial to incorporate a daily exercise program into their lives. Often exercise, such as jumping on a mini trampoline, is less strenuous and can be done throughout the whole pregnancy if it is started early in the pregnancy. This has been know to make the childbirth much easier.

CONCEPTION

Childless couples wishing to conceive, have had dramatic success when both the husband and wife have taken Formula #28 and large doses of Vitamin E. These help to strengthen the reproductive orgains of both sexes. The wife may also take Formula #13.

BEGINNING PREGNANCY

Red Raspberry taken as tea or in capsules should be started as soon as the mother discovers that she is pregnant, and should be continued throughout the pregnancy. Formula #3 should also be taken early in the pregnancy as it helps provide energy and contains all of the vitamins and minerals that the body needs. It contains Alfalfa, which is rich in all of the trace minerals, Kelp, which will help keep the weight off the middle and hip area, and is a natural source of iodine, and Dandelion, which acts as a natural diuretic and will provide natural iron for the blood. This Formula has been used historically to help prevent birth defects. The mother should use a good natural multivitamin-mineral supplement.

CAUTIONS:

The following herbs should not be used during early pregnancy: Aloe Vera, Don Quai, Pennyroyal, and Rue. Harsh laxatives should also be avoided, as well as herbs that contain steroids or hormones.

MORNING SICKNESS

This can be due to a deficiency of Vitamin B complex in the diet. Often, however vitamin B cannot be tolerated.

Red Raspberry tea or Peppermint tea are often used to help overcome the nausea. Alfalfa and Peppermint tea can be taken together for good results. (See Formula #11) Catnip Tea, Ginger Tea, or other pleasant tasting herbs can also be used to help settle the stomach. There are herbal oil combinations that can also be used. Sometimes it helps to take small, frequent meals instead of three larger ones.

MISCARRIAGE

False Unicorn and Lobelia are best and should be used together.

TOXEMIA

Formula #4 will help purify the blood. Alfalfa, Comfrey, Red Raspberry, Yellow Dock, Chlorophyll and Vitamin C are also used for toxemia.

LAST SIX WEEKS

Formula #5 is very high in calcium and silicon which are important in building good bones and teeth in the baby and providing the mother with sufficient calcium for herself. It should be taken in abundance, especially during the last month of pregnancy. Formula #6 is used during this last period of help make the labor and delivery easier. It will help strengthen the uterus and female organs. Blue Cohosh is also added at this time to help the labor process.

LABOR AND DELIVERY

The herbs in the previous section should be continued. More Blue Cohosh may be taken. Vitamin E will decrease the need for oxygen and help breathing during labor. Corn Silk can promote labor if it stops. Red Raspberry is essential during labor. It coordinates the uterine contractions often making labor shorter.

FALSE LABOR

Catnip tea and Blue Cohosh have been used to stop false labor. Walking sometimes will help.

RETAINED PLACENTA

Licorice, Mistletoe, Thyme, Red Raspberry, and Slippery Elm have all been used to help release a retained placenta.

POST PARTUM & AFTERPAIN

Nutmeg contains the Alkaloid, Erganovine which will contract the uterus and help stop bleeding after childbirth. Cayenne and Bayberry are also used to slow the bleeding. If the bleeding is serious, then Yarrow, Mistletoe, and Corn Silk are used. Chlorophyll and Shepherd's Purse both contain Vitamin K which will help the blood to clot.

B. BABIES AND CHILDREN

Powdered herbs can be put in applesauce, honey, or 1/2 teaspoon of molasses. They can also be made into teas, or capsules can be inserted in the baby's rectum.

1. Colic — Catnip, Fennel, Peppermint or any combination of these three in a tea. Use no sugar as it may cause more colic.

2. Constipation — Licorice tea. The nursing mother can pass herbs to her baby that will also help.

3. Cradle Cap — Olive Oil or Vitamin E on the head and brush gently.

4. Diaper Rash — Mullein Leaf, Slippery Elm (Used internally in juice) or apply as paste. Garlic water or oil can be applied externally. Also Vitamin E can be used. Powdered Golden Seal or Comfrey can be added to the baby powder. The nursing mother can take Vitamins A, B, and C.

5. Diarrhea — Slippery Elm enema (1/2 teaspoon to 1 cup water) Red Raspberry tea (drink or use as an enema) Fresh apple juice, banana, brown rice water, or carob can also be given. Slippery Elm or Carob can also be added to boiled - milk.

6. Dry Skin	Olive Oil instead of commercial baby oil is good.
7. Ear Infection	Garlic oil, Mullein oil, Lobelia extract or Combination "C" extract may be dropped in the ear. Ice packs can be used to disperse the blood flow around the ears and ease the aching. Vitamin C and Formula #18 can be used. Golden Seal capsule in the rectum.
8. Fever	Catnip tea enema, Red Raspberry tea, or Peppermint tea.
9. Hyperactivity	Lobelia, and Formulas #5 and #23 are good. Vitamin B complex and multiple mineral supplements are beneficial. Avoid all artificial flavoring and food coloring.
10. Loss of Appetite	Camomile tea or Peppermint tea.
11. Pinworms	Camomile tea. Raisins soaked in Senna Tea for older children.
12. Restlessness	Hops tea. 1 teaspoon of Lobelia extract rubbed on the back will help. A few drops of the extract on the tongue will relax the baby.
13. Teething	Rub Lobelia extract on the gums. White Oak Bark tea can also be given. Aloe Vera gel or Peppermint oil can also be rubbed on the gums.
14. Yeast Infection	Yogurt or acidophilus is used. Garlic oil or water can be used.

C. NURSING

Blessed Thistle (cold), Chlorophyll, Fennel, Alfalfa, Red Raspberry, or Marshmallow (warm) will bring in good rich milk. This will sustain the baby longer and help him sleep through the night at an earlier age.

Parsley, Kelp, and Sage will help dry up the milk when the mother is ready to quit nursing.

For caked breasts, use Poke Root packs.

If the baby has an infection, the mother can take Vitamin C and Formula #18 or other Vitamins and herbs and the baby will receive them through the milk.

CAUTION: If the nursing mother is taking too many cleansing herbs it may cause colic or diarrhea in the baby.

HERBS THAT CONTAIN STEROIDS

The following herbs contain steroids which may have a hormonal effect on the body and should be used with caution during pregnancy. Children and nursing mothers should also be cautious of these herbs. They should only be used when necessary and for short periods of time.

Black Cohosh	Don Quai	Sarsaparilla
Blessed Thistle	False Unicorn	Saw Palmetto
Blue Cohosh	Ginseng	Squaw Vine
Cramp Bark	Licorice	Wild Yam
Damiana	Pennyroyal	Yarrow

Chapter 6
VITAMIN AND MINERAL SOURCES

Vitamin A	Alfalfa, Burdock, Cayenne, Comfrey, Dandelion, Garlic, kelp, Marshmallow, Papaya, Parsley, Pokeweed, Raspberry, Red Clover, Safflower, Watercress, Yellow Dock.
Vitamin B1 (Thiamine)	Cayenne, Dandelion, Fenugreek, Kelp, Parsley, Raspberry.
Vitamin B2 (Riboflavin)	Alfalfa, Burdock, Dandelion, Fenugreek, Kelp, Parsley, Safflower, Watercress.
Vitamin B3 (Niacin)	Alfalfa, Burdock, Dandelion, Fenugreek, Kelp, Parsley, Sage.
Vitamin B6 (Pyridoxine)	Alfalfa, Chlorophyll
Vitamin B12 (Cyanocobalamin)	Alfalfa, Chlorophyll, Don Quai, Kelp.
Vitamin C	Alfalfa, Burdock, Boneset, Catnip, Cayenne, Chickweed, Dandelion, Garlic, Hawthorn, Horseradish, Kelp, Lobelia, Parsley, Plantain, Pokeweed, Papaya, Raspberry, Rose Hips, Shepherd's Purse, Strawberry, Watercress, Yellow Dock.
Vitamin D	Alfalfa, Chlorophyll, Watercress.
Vitamin E	Alfalfa, Dandelion, Don Quai, Kelp, Raspberry, Rose Hips, Watercress.
Vitamin G	Alfalfa, Cayenne, Dandelion, Gotu Kola, Kelp.
Vitamin K	Alfalfa, Chlorophyll, Plantain, Shepherd's Purse.
Vitamin P (Rutin)	Dandelion, Rose Hips, Rue.

Vitamin T	Plantain
Vitamin U (For Peptic Ulcers)	Alfalfa, Chlorophyll
Aluminum	Alfalfa, Chlorophyll
Calcium	Alfalfa, Blue Cohosh, Camomile, Cayenne, Chlorophyll, Comfrey, Dandelion, Horsetail, Irish Moss, Kelp, Mistletoe, Nettle, Parsley, Plantain, Pokeweed, Raspberry, Rose Hips, Shepherd's Purse, Strawberry Fruit, Yarrow, Yellow Dock.
Chlorine	Alfalfa, Dandelion, Kelp, Parsley, Raspberry.
Copper	Kelp, Parsley.
Fluorine	Alfalfa, Garlic.
Iodine	Black Walnut, Dulse, Garlic, Irish Moss, Kelp, Sarsaparilla.
Iron	Alfalfa, Burdock, Blue Cohosh, Cayenne, Chlorophyll, Dandelion, Dulse, Kelp, Mullein, Nettle, Parsley, Pokeweed, Rhubarb, Rose Hips, Strawberry Fruit, Yarrow, Yellow Dock.
Lithium	Kelp.
Magnesium	Alfalfa, Blue Cohosh, Cayenne, Dandelion, Irish Moss, Kelp, Mistletoe, Mullein, Peppermint, Primrose, Raspberry, Willow, Wintergreen.
Manganese	Kelp.
Phosphorus	Alfalfa, Blue Cohosh, Caraway, Cayenne, Chickweed, Dandelion, Garlic, Irish Moss, Kelp, Licorice, Parsley, Purslane, Pokeweed, Raspberry, Rose Hips, Watercress, Yellow Dock.
Potassium	Alfalfa, Blue Cohosh, Birch, Borage, Camomile, Coltsfoot, Comfrey, Centaury, Dandelion, Dulse, Eyebright, Fennel, Irish Moss, Kelp, Mistletoe, Mullein, Nettle, Papaya, Parsley, Peppermint, Plantain, Primrose, Raspberry, Shepherd's Purse, Strawberry Fruit, White Oak Bark, Wintergreen, Yarrow.
Selenium	Kelp.

Silicon	Alfalfa, Blue Cohosh, Burdock, Horsetail, Kelp, Nettle, Oat Straw, Strawberry Fruit.
Sodium	Alfalfa, Dandelion, Dulse, Fennel, Irish Moss, Kelp, Mistletoe, Parsley, Shepherd's Purse, Strawberry Fruit, Willow, Yarrow.
Sulfur	Alfalfa, Burdock, Cayenne, Coltsfoot, Eyebright, Fennel, Garlic, Irish Moss, Kelp, Mullein, Nettle, Parsley, Plantain, Raspberry, Sage, Shepherd's Purse, Strawberry Fruit, Thyme, Yarrow.
Zinc	Kelp, Marshmallow.
Trace Minerals	Alfalfa, Kelp.

Chapter 7

POISONOUS PLANTS

Autumn Crocus . . . . Bulb
Azaleas . . . . All parts
Black Locust . . . . Bark, Sprouts, Foliage
Buttercup . . . . All parts
Daffodil . . . . Bulb
Elderberry . . . . Shoots, Leaves, Bark
Fox Glove . . . . Leaves
Hyacinth . . . . Bulb
Iris . . . . Underground stems
Jack-in-the-Pulpit . . . . All parts
Jimson Weed . . . . All parts
Larkspur . . . . Young plants, Seeds
Lily-of-the-Valley . . . . Leaves, Flowers
May Apple . . . . Apple, Foliage, Roots
Mistletoe . . . . Berries
Monkshood . . . . Fleshy roots
Moon Seed . . . . Berries
Narcissus . . . . Bulb
Night Shade . . . . All parts
Oaks . . . . Foliage, Acorns
Oleander . . . . Leaves, Branches
Poinsetta . . . . Leaves
Poison Hemlock . . . . All parts
Poison Ivy . . . . All parts
Potato . . . . Leaves
Rhubarb . . . . Leaves, Blade
Star of Bethlehem . . . . Bulb
Water Hemlock . . . . All parts
Wild & Cultivated Cherries . . . . . Twigs, Foliage
Wisteria . . . . Seeds, Pods

See *Nature's Medicine Chest* by LeArta Moulton
for colored pictures of these herbs.

Chapter 8
CLEANSING

In illness, the body has many ways of ridding itself of toxins. Mucous is expelled from sinuses in the form of a runny nose, from the lungs by coughing. Toxins are eliminated through the colon by diarrhea, and the stomach, by vomiting.

This is all part of the cleansing process. We can help this process by diet, fasting, enemas, exercise, and a healthy mental attitude.

DIET

The purpose of a cleanse is to elminate excessive mucous and toxins from the body. Animal protein, white flour, and white sugar are all very mucuous forming, therefore slowing down the cleansing process.

Research indicates that the intestines in carniverous animals are shorter than those in herbiverous animals. The meat must pass through the colon quickly or it putrifies, forming toxins that are assimilated into the body. The human intestine is longer than the intestine of carniverous animals, thus indicating that the main portion of his diet should be vegetables and fruits.

The diet should consist mainly of fresh fruits and vegetables, nuts, and seeds. Vegetables should be eaten raw whenever possible, but if they are cooked, they should be steamed just until tender, or baked.

Vitamin and mineral supplements may be added to the diet, but should be from a natural source, as some people have allergic or chemical reactions to synthetic vitamins.

BASIC NUTRITIONAL GUIDELINES

Avoid refined and processed foods.

Protein: Use meat sparingly — especially red meat, and never after 1 p.m. Fresh fish and organically grown chicken are the best.

Dairy:	Cheese, Butter, Yogurt, and other dairy products should be made from raw milk. Pasteurization destroys enzymes, amino acids, and vitamins, causing excess mucous in the body. Raw goat's milk is easier to digest than raw cow's milk.
Eggs:	Farm fresh eggs that have been laid by chickens in their natural habitat are more nutritious and more easily assimilated.
Nuts & Grains:	Nuts and grains are good foods but due to sensitivities that most people have to them, sprouting is often recommended.
Fruits &:	May be used freely but should be whole, and unpeeled whenever possible. When cooking, some water should be used as dry cooking destroys many nutrients. One of the best ways to cook potatoes and apples is in a covered glass baking dish at 350° for 1 1/2 hours with approximately 1/4 inch water in bottom. The remaining water should be used as it is full of the water soluble vitamins. Soups are nutritious because the nutrients that are cooked out of the food are retained in the liuqid.
Water:	Plenty of fresh water that is free from chemical threatment such as fluoride or chlorine. At least half the body weight in ounces should be taken each day.
Oils & Fats:	The only ones to be used are olive oil & raw butter.
Sweetners:	Eliminate all sugar from the diet and substitute raw honey, molasses, and pure maple syrup. Fructose may be used sparingly.
Salt:	Use a good, natural salt such as rock salt or sea salt.

TWO PHASE BALANCING DIET

This two phase diet has been used successfully by Dr. Dan Lafferty to bring the body into a balanced state where it can tolerate allergy-causing foods.

PHASE I (non-reactive foods)

This phase of the diet is to prime the system and to bring the pH to 7.5 for 2 days in succession (usually about 5 days). There may be some unusual changes take place in the first few days, such as — anxiety, depression, intolerance, or possibly even a rash.

Foods to be used in Phase I:

- Potatoes: (preferably red, not sweet or yams)
- Root Vegetables: (carrots, beets, turnips, rutabagas (not onions)
- Leaves & Stems: beet greens, celery, chard, lettuce, cabbage
- Fruits: Apples, pears, peaches, apricots, plums, nectarines, and cherries. (Do not eat core)
- Herbs: Spearmint, peppermint, and comfrey (tea)
- Oil: Only Olive Oil is used.
- Salt: Natural rock or sea salt.
     Cinnamon and apple cider vinegar can be used occasionally for flavoring.

Cooking of foods is very important. It begins the digestion process and reduces stress on the body and increases nutrient assimilation.

See nutritional guidelines for directions on how to cook.

Olive oil is an important part of the diet and should be increased as needed for hunger and lack of energy. Use generously.

These Phase I foods can be eaten in any combination. It is necessary to eat some food every 2 to 3 hours for accurate urine samples. (1st morning sample exception)

BREAKFAST: Steam 6 to 8 carrots until tender than add 8 to 10 potatoes, previously baked and approximately 1 cup olive oil. Mash to desired consistency and salt to taste. (If you make a large quantity, it can be refrigerated and reheated for other meals — we call this "Now & Later." A helping of this plus some comfrey tea is a good breakfast.

SNACK: Fresh Fruit

LUNCH: Sauted potatoes, boiled greens, and tea. Do not fry but stir in the olive oil until warm. "Now & Later." With salad is another variation.

SNACK: Fresh Fruit

DINNER:	Hot baked potato with olive oil poured on like gravy. Green salad with olive oil & vinegar dressing, vegetable, and tea. If you desire, a baked apple with cinnamon.

PHASE II (Reactive Foods)

After your pH has stayed at 7.5 for 2 successive days, this phase is started. There are 5 foods that represent this group. They are gradually added to the non-reactive food group above.

Raw milk
Raw butter
Farm fresh eggs
Raw Honey
Oat Groats (not rolled)

These are used in addition to the phase I diet for 3 days and then go back on just the Phase I diet for 2 days. Continue this until your pH stays at 7.5 for the 3 days you are on the Phase II diet. It is often beneficial to go on the Phase I diet at least 2 days each month.

There are 2 rules for foods not on this list:
  1. Don't eat them often — have them for special occasions
  2. Enjoy them when you eat them.
A Healthy body can easily stand the negative effects of eating a treat on occasion, but it needs to be the exception rather than the rule as it has come to be so much today.

FASTING

Fasting is necessary to help the body heal and throw off diseases, parasites, growths, mucous, and poisonous toxins.
There are several methods of fasting:

Mild food, juice, fruits and nuts, broth, water, or total abstinence from food and water.

We do not recommend total abstinence, nor do we recommend fasting for long periods of time without supervision from a doctor.
Studies have shown that people who fast and are deprived of their daily food intake will break down and digest their own diseased, damaged, aged, or dead cells. During this time, new healthy cells are being produced to replace the diseased ones.
Since vitamins and minerals interfere with the cleansing process, they should be discontinued while fasting. Herbs may be used as they help to cleanse the body and regulate the glands.
Juice should be from fresh fruits and vegetables diluted with distilled water. (If these are unavailable, unsweetened canned or

frozen juices may be used.) At least eight glasses of liquid should be taken during the day. The first three days are the hardest, but the most benefit comes after the third day. The fast is broken when the body experiences extreme hunger.

Each day of the fast should include:

Cleansing enema	Distilled or spring water
Dry brush massage	Herb teas
Hot and cold shower	Diluted juices
Walking or other exercise	Vegetable broth
At least a one hour rest	

Vegetable Broth

Chop or grate the following into 1½ quarts of boiling water:

2 large red potatoes (skins included)
3 stalks celery
3 medium beets
4 carrots

Add any of the following vegetables: cabbage, turnips, turnip tops, beet tops, onions.

Season with any of your favorite herbs — Rosemary, Sage, Thyme, Parsley, Oregano, Basil, Cayenne.

Cover and simmer 45 minutes. When slightly cool, blend in the blender and drink warm.

Anyone can fast, but it takes a determined person to break it. It should be broken properly over a period of three to four days. Remember to eat lightly and to chew your food well.

1st day:	1 fruit for breakfast Vegetable salad for lunch
2nd day:	Same as 1st day only add vegetable soup for dinner 2 more fruits throughout the day
3rd day:	Add larger portions of fruit and salad Nuts and soured milk products Baked potato or squash Bread and butter Soup
4th day:	Start back on mild food.

GREEN DRINK

A cleansing, nutritious drink made from herbs, is what we call the "green drink." Many herbs can be used, but we find that if you use no more than four at a time it tastes better. Here are a few ideas for the drink.

Put fresh Pineapple or unsweetened Pineapple Juice in the blender then add any of the following:

Burdock, Carrot tops, **Celery,** Chard, **Comfrey,** Dandelion, Marshmallow, **Parsley**, Plantain, Radish tops, Raspberry Leaves, Sprouts, Wheat Grass.

Blend and strain, make fresh each day.

CAUTION: Do not use Potato Leaves or Rhubarb Leaves.

DRY BRUSH MASSAGE

Dirt, dust, pollution, and inactivity cause the pores to get congested. Since the skin is the largest eliminative organ of the body, if these pores get clogged, the skin will become either too dry or too oily. Brushing the body either with a body brush or loofa helps to open up the pores so the toxins can escape.

EXERCISE

Since illness is caused by blocked circulation, exercise is important to increase the cirulation. It is usually needed the most when you feel the least like doing it.

Exercise will help move the toxins through the lymphatic system and out of the body through the colon, kidneys, skin, and eliminative organs. Jogging is a common means of exercise if done in moderation and with proper supportive shoes.

However, in his article, "Jogging Can Kill You" Dr. J. E. Schmidt indicates that jogging can be injurious to the body as it often jars the organs and skeletal system. Jumping and running are better if they are done on some soft, or flexible surface, such as a trampoline. There are some units designed especially for this purpose already on the market. This will help the cirulcation and cause one to breathe deeply, which most of us fail to do.

May I quote Dr. Paavo Airola from his lecture in September 1975. "It is better to eat junk food and exercise than to eat good food without exercising."

PERSPIRATION

Perspiration helps rid the body of toxins. Hot baths, and the use of certain herbs in the bath water will increase the circulation and open the pores. Any of the following may be used:

1. Add 3 to 4 tablespoons of ginger to a tub of warm water.
2. Add 1 cup vinegar and 1/2 cup salt to a tub of warm water. Sit in the tub until perspiration ceases.
3. Put enough mineral water in a pan to cover the feet. Soak them for 1/2 hour.

Take a cool shower after each hot bath to close the pores.

To eliminate toxins faster, sip several glasses of water while in the tub.

CAUTION: Some people get dizzy while sitting in the tub, so we suggest that there be some type of ventilation or a cool cloth to use on the forehead.

If a person has a fever, do not use hot water. Cool water will help bring the fever down quicker.

ENEMAS

During a fast, the eliminative organs are used extensively in order to remove the concentrated wastes. This is why it is important to take enemas. When the colon is congested, toxins are absorbed back into the system manifesting themselves as fever, earache, sore throat, headache, or any other illness.

There are many types of enemas but we have used the following with excellent results:

Cayenne: Used to stimulate the liver, kidneys, spleen, and pancreas. It will also help stop bleeding. Add 1/2 teaspoon cayenne to a bag of water. CAUTION: If a person has serious problems in the colon, this could cause a burning sensation.

Garlic: Used for a general cleanser and to help elminate parasites. Blend 1 or 2 garlic buds for each bag, in 1 quart of water. Strain. Add enough water to fill the bag. Do this three times.

Catnip: Use for fever, colic, and contagious diseases. It is very relaxing to the whole system. Make a tea of 2 Tablespoons catnip in a quart of water. Strain. Add enough water to fill the bag.

114

Mineral Water: 1/2 cup to bag of water. Use for general cleansing.

Slippery Elm: Used for diarrhea, colitis, and hemorrhoids. Put 1 Tablespoon powder in blender with 1 pint of water. Add enough water to fill the bag.

White Oak Bark: Used for hemorrhoids, colitis, and it is very healing. Make tea with 2 Tablespoons White Oak Bark. Add enough water to fill the bag.

When available, distilled water should be used. The knee-chest position helps the water to go through the colon better. The first bag should be warm water, as it relaxes the colon and the water is expelled faster. The second and third bags should be slightly cool water to stimulate the peristaltic action. The water is retained longer to break loose the toxins and pockets of decayed matter.

Lubricate the end of the tube with vitamin E, or petroleum jelly. Insert it just inside the rectum. As the water runs in, you can slowly insert the tube further. Never go further than 18 to 24 inches, and only as long as it moves rather easily. Don't ever force the tube in further.

The moment you have a slight cramp, or feel a need to expel, remove the tube and relax for elimination. Don't hold the water longer, as this only balloons out the colon.

Continue to do this until you have used 3 bags. For children, adjust this amount according to age. Always take acidophilus, yogurt, buttermilk, or kefir to replace the natural bacteria in the colon after taking enemas.

Chapter 9
HERBAL AID FOR EMERGENCIES

ASTHMA

For an acute attack, put several drops of Lobelia Extract in the mouth and it will relax the throat. Usually the colon needs to be cleaned out to help the whole system.

BEE STINGS

Apply ice until swelling and pain are gone. Honey helps pull out the stinger and neutralizes the poison. Mud or Redmond Clay can be used if Honey is not available.

BLEEDING

Golden Seal, or Plantain applied directly on wound. Take either of above internally. If there is heavy bleeding, take Cayenne in hot water until it stops. (See Hemorrhage) Cayenne can be applied externally on small wounds.

BURNS

Apply ice water and keep cloth wet and cold until pain leaves. Apply Aloe Vera on burn and also take internally. Formula #26 mixed with either Vitamin E or mineral water makes an excellent poultice. Always apply vitamin E on burn before applying poultice. Honey applied on burn also helps.

COUGH

1. 1/4 teaspoon each of Cayenne and Ginger.
   1 Tablespoon each of Honey and Vinegar.
   Add 2 Tablespoons hot water, mix and take by spoon.
2. Mix juice from 1/2 lemon with 2 Tablespoons Honey and take every 15 minutes.
3. Licorice Tea or Lobelia Extract can be taken.

CROUP

Cleanse the Colon with a Catnip Tea Enema. A few drops of Lobelia Extract by mouth helps to relax. Eucalyptus Oil may be used in the steamer.

DIARRHEA

Any of the following may be used:
   1/2 teaspoon Nutmeg several times a day.
   1 Tablespoon of Slippery Elm in bag of water as an enema.
   Raspberry Leaf Tea as enema or internally.
   1 teaspoon of Carob Powder in 1 cup boiled milk.
   1 teaspoon whole cloves steeped in 1 quart water used as tea.

EARACHE

Take a cleansing enema to clean out the colon. Oil of Mullein, Garlic Oil, or Lobelia Extract in the ear. Ice pack on ear to help constrict blood vessels. B & B Tincture or "C" Extract drops in ear. (Chapter 1)

FEVER

Take a Catnip Tea Enema to break loose congestion. 1,000 milligrams of Vitamin C each hour throughout the day. Juices. Tepid ginger or vinegar and salt bath. See section on perspiration in chapter 8. Calcium also helps to bring the fever down.

FLU

(Formula #14) for intestinal flu.
Cleansing enema, vitamin C, juices.
Raspberry Tea, Echinacea are both good for flu.
4 Teaspoons each of Catnip and Peppermint in 1 quart boiling water. Steep and drink. Go to bed and perspire.

GALL STONES

1. 3 Day Gall Stone Cleanse:
   1st day: Apple juice all day. Before going to bed take 1 cup olive oil and 1/2 cup lemon juice.
   2nd day: Enema in morning and then same as first day.
   3rd day: Same as second day.
2. Alternate Cleanse: Two days of apple juice and on third morning,
   take 1 cup olive oil and 1 cup lemon juice followed by a garlic enema.
   When the stones are passed, they are usually a dark green or black in color.

3. Overnight Gallstone Cleanse

    1 pint olive oil

    1/2 pint lemon juice

It is all right to eat an early breakfast. Take an enema or a colonic after eating. Fast during the day until 2 hours before retiring. Take 2 oz. of the oil and 1 oz. of the juice every 15 minutes. Go to bed lying on the right side with a pillow under the hips. This will concentrate the "brew" in the gall bladder. Early the next morning when you have the urge to eliminate, the stones should pass.

HEMORRHOIDS

Cut a piece of raw, red potato the size of your little finger and apply vitamin E. Insert this in rectum at night. This helps take away the pain and reduce the swelling. Take a White Oak Bark tea enema — 1 Tablespoon of the herb to a bag of water.

KIDNEY STONES

2 Tablespoons lemon juice in water, and Formula #19 taken every half hour usually relieves the pain and will help the stones to pass.

SORE THROAT

Take an enema. Swab the throat with glycerine and iodine. Put an onion pack around the neck. (See Chapter 1; see also TONSILLITIS.) Wring a cloth out of strong salt water solution and put it around the neck with a plastic cover to keep the moisture in and the pillow dry.

Vitamins: A, C

TONSILLITIS

Take a garlic enema. 1,000 milligrams vitamin C every hour with 2 capsules of Formula #18. Swab or gargle with glycerine and iodine. (Use enough iodine in the glycerine to make it a deep amber color.)

The enema cleans out the colon so the infection has a place to go, the vitamin C and Formula #18 help to fight infection, and the glycerine and iodine help to take the swelling down.

Cayenne may be used as a gargle.

Usually one day is sufficient, but sometimes it will take longer.

BIBLIOGRAPHY

Adams, Ruth and Frank Murray. *All You Should Know About Health Foods.* New York: Larchmont Books, 1975.

Airola, Paavo. *How To Get Well.* Phoenix, Arizona: Health Plus Publishers, 1974.

Clegg, Bud, ed. *Herbalist,* Provo, Utah: Bi-World Publishers, 1976.

Dickey, Esther, *Passport to Survival.* Salt Lake City, Utah: Bookcraft Publishers, 1969.

Gathercoal, Edmund N. PhG, PhM, *Pharmacognosy,* Philadelphia, Pa. Lea & Febiger, 1936.

Griffin, LaDean. *No Side Effects,* Provo, Utah: Bi-World Publishers, 1975.

Harris, Ben Charles. *Eat the Weeds.* New Canaan, Connecticut: Keats Publishing, Inc., 1973.

Hawley, Don, ed. *Life and Health National Health Journal.* Washington, D. C.: Review and Herald Publishing Association, 1973.

Hylton, William H., ed. *The Rodale Herb Book.* Emmaus, Pennsylvania: Rodale Press, 1975.

Kloss, Jethro. *Back to Eden.* Santa Barbara, California: Lifeline Books, 1975.

Kordel, Lelord. *Natural Folk Remedies.* New York: Manor Books, Inc., 1976.

Levy, Juliette de Bairacli. *Common Herbs For Natural Health,* New York, Schocken Books, 1979.

Lust, John. *The Herb Book.* Simi Valley, California: Benedict Lust Publications, 1974.

Mindell, Earl, *The Vitamin Bible,* Warner Community Co.

Moulton, LeArta. *Nature's Medicine Chest.* Provo, Utah: The Gluten Co., 1975.

Stille, Alfred, M.D. LL.D. et al., *The National Dispensatory.* Philadelphia, Pa.

Taub, Harold J., ed. *Let's Live.* Los Angeles, California: Oxford Industries, Inc., 1976.

Weiner, Michael A. *Earth Medicine — Earth Foods.* New York, Collier Books, 1972.

INDEX

*Health problems are listed in capital letters.
The bold numbers indicate pages with major information.*

BOILS 15, 16, 18, 21, 22, 24, 25, 31, 33-35, 39, 41, 42, 47, 49, **63**

BREASTS 38, 41, 63, **73**, 102

Brigham Tea **17**, 60-62, 65, 66, 73, 76, 77, 81, 85, 91, 92

BRONCHITIS 16, 19-27, 31-34, 37-44, 46, 50, 52, 54, 56, **63**

BRUISES 22, 24, 26, 28, 31, 33, 34, 36, 40, 42, 45, 47, **63**

Buchu **18**, 62, 69, 81, 90, 91, 96, 97

Buckthorn **18**, 67, 75, 78, 81, 82, 88, 89, 91, 92, 97

Burdock **18**, 58-66, 72, 75, 76, 78, 81-84, 86-89, 91-95, 97, 98

BURNS 14, 18, 21, 22, 28, 31, 34, 37, 42, **64, 116**

BURSITIS 14, 18, 21, 22, 32-35, 45, 47-49, **64**

C

Calcium **49**

Camomile **19**, 60-63, 65-69, 71-78, 80-82, 85, 87, 88, 90, 93, 95, 98

CANCER 21, 24, 25, 27, 28, 31, 36, 38, 42, 43, 49, 50, **64**

CANKER (see MOUTH SORES)

Capsicum (see CAYENNE)

Cascara Sagrada **19**, 67-69, 71, 75, 78, 82, 87, 93

CATARACTS (see EYES) 21, 25, 51

Catnip **20**, 63, 65, 66, 67, 69-71, 73-76, 79-81, 84-89, 93, 96, 98, 114

Cayenne 11, **20**, 58-63, 65-69, 71, 72, 74-79, 81-86, 91-95, 97, 98, 114

Chaparral **21**, 58, 59-65, 68, 69, 72, 76, 80, 81, 88, 90-92, 95, 97, 98

CHICKENPOX **65**

Chickweed **21**, 58, 59, 61, 63-65, 67, 69, 76-78, 80, 81, 83, 86, 87, 90-95, 98

CHILDBIRTH 17, 23, 32, 35, 37, 39, 42, **49, 65**

CHILDHOOD DISEASES 15, 17-20, 27, 28, 33, 34, 38-41, 43, 44, 47, 49, 50, 53, **65**

Chlorophyll **22,** 58, 59, 61, 62, 65, 67, 69 71-74, 76, 78, 79, 81, 82, 84, 86, 89, 93-95

CIRCULATION 15, 16, 20, 21, 27-31, 38, 40, 53, **65**

CLEANSING 18, 21, 22, 24, 33, 39, 43, 47, 49, **50,** 54, 57, **66, 108**

COLDS 15, 17, 19, 20, 22, 26-28, 32, 37, 39-41, 44, 47, 49, **50,** 52, 53, 56, **66**

COLIC 17, 19, 26, 37, 44, 45, 47, 51, **66, 101**

COLITIS 19, 20, 22, 26-28, 32, 33, 35-38, 42, 44, 49, 50, **57, 66**

COLON 14, 15, 19, 21, 22, 25-27, 31, 34, 35, 38, 42-44, 47, 49, **50,** 57, **67**

Concentrated Herbs 13

Comfrey 12, **22,** 59-64, 66-72, 74-81, 83, 84, 86, 91-96, 98

CONCEPTION **99**

CONSTIPATION 14, 15, 17-19, 21, 23, 24, 28, 33, 34, 38, 39, 42, 44, 49, 50, 55, 57, **67,** 101

CONVULSIONS & EPILEPSY 16, 17, 20, 24, 26, 28, 30, 31, 33, 34, 36-38, 41, 44-46, 49, 55, 57, **67**

Corn Silk **23,** 62, 65, 75, 77, 81, 88, 90, 96, 98

COUGH 16, 19, 20, 22, 25-31, 33-38, 41-43, 46, 52, 56, **68, 116**

Couch Grass **23,** 62, 63, 67, 75, 81, 82, 88, 98

CRADLE CAP **101**

Cramp Bark **23,** 81, 84, 85, 87, 96, 103

CRAMPS 14, 16, 17, 19-24, 26, 27, 32, 37, 40, 42, 48, 49, 52, 55, **68**

CROUP 19, 20, 25, 27, 33, 34, 43, 44, 50, **69, 117**

CUTS (see WOUNDS)

123

125